Psychodermatology

Psychodermatology covers all aspects of how the mind and body interact in relation to the onset and progression of various skin disorders. This book is the first text written by a multidisciplinary team of psychiatrists, psychologists, child specialists and dermatologists for all the health professionals who treat patients with skin problems. They cover a broad range of issues affecting these patients, including: stigma, coping, relationships, psychological treatments, the impact on children, psychosocial comorbidity, psychoneuroimmunology, quality of life and psychological treatments.

CARL WALKER is a health psychologist with wide practical and research experience in the field of psychodermatology. He has published widely in health-based psychology journals on the psychological and social aspects of skin disease and is co-author of *Understanding Skin Problems*, a guide written to help skin disease patients address the challenges they face when coping with the different aspects of their illness. He also currently co-ordinates an EU-funded European-wide research programme assessing risk factors for depression in primary care.

LINDA PAPADOPOULOS is a chartered health and counselling psychologist. She has published widely in the field of medical psychology and psychodermatology and gives specialist lectures around the world on working with clients with disfigurement and skin disease. Her research is often featured in the media and her publications such as *Psychological Approaches to Dermatology* and *Understanding Skin Problems* are important contributions in the field of dermatology and disfigurement.

Psychodermatology

Edited by

Carl Walker

and

Linda Papadopoulos

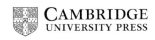

CAMBRIDGE
UNIVERSITY PRESS

CAMBRIDGE UNIVERSITY PRESS
Cambridge, New York, Melbourne, Madrid, Cape Town, Singapore, São Paulo

CAMBRIDGE UNIVERSITY PRESS
The Edinburgh Building, Cambridge CB2 2RU, UK

Published in the United States of America by Cambridge University Press, New York
www.cambridge.org
Information on this title: www.cambridge.org/9780521542296

First published 2005

Printed in the United Kingdom at the University Press, Cambridge

A catalog record for this publication is available from the British Library

Library of Congress Cataloging in Publication data

ISBN-13   978-0-521-54229-6 paperback
ISBN-10   0-521-54229-4 paperback

Contents

9   Research methodology in quality of life assessment   116

Andrew Finlay

Preface

When considering the impact of skin disease, many people fail to realise just how important the psychological aspects can be. Skin disease is often considered to be 'only cosmetic' by many medical professionals and lay-people alike, but unlike most internal illnesses, skin disease is often immediately visible to others. It is for this reason that traditional views do not account for the often profound psychological impact that it can exert on those affected. Skin disease can affect the quality of life, self-esteem and body image, as well as the way patients live their day-to-day lives. Furthermore, the way that skin disease affects a person often has no relation to traditional conceptualisations of medical severity. To truly understand the effect, we need to understand the person behind the condition. Through the course of our work we have encountered individuals whose skin disease covers the majority of the surface of their skin but whose social and psychological functioning were unaffected by the condition. Conversely, individuals with the smallest of lesions in non-visible areas have been so affected by their condition that occupational, social and sexual interactions have fallen prey to their functional inability to cope with their condition. The unique nature of skin disease has the potential to make it both the easiest or most difficult disease to suffer and how a person copes and adapts to the challenges presented is due to a great number of factors. Recent years have seen a considerable increase in research concerned with the psychological effects of skin disease on patients and their families, and we are beginning to appreciate the degree to which a variety of problems confront both patients and their wider social networks.

The question of what exactly is psychodermatology is one that should be addressed at the start of this text so that we understand the direction with which we, as health professionals, approach the topic. Psychodermatology is as much an ethos as a discipline; a professional, clinical and research-orientated awareness, and acceptance of the psychological and social implications of dermatological conditions and this text is an important contribution to the field of psychodermatology, not only because of its content but because of the readership that we hope to target. This book was designed to give us a better understanding of the ways in which health professionals can be maximally effective in addressing the different elements that matter to skin disease sufferers of all ages. As such, it has been written for a broad range of readers comprising not only researchers who work in the area of skin disease but the range of professionals who come into contact with skin disease patients and their families, including dermatologists, dermatology nurses, psychologists, psychiatrists and general practitioners. The chapters in this volume offer a guided tour through the key areas of the subject, discussing in detail the biological, psychological and social implications of dermatology, and we would like to think that this provides professionals with a reference framework for the different factors involved in living with skin disease.

We feel that there should be a greater collaboration between clinicians and researchers in order to improve both the quality of research and the quality of clinical care that patients receive, and this volume highlights just why this is so crucial.

Above all, we hope that this text will stimulate professionals working in the field of dermatology to explore their supportive communication and increase awareness regarding the difficulties that patients with skin disease can face. One of the great problems facing those with skin disease is the trivialisation and minimisation of the associated difficulties and distress and if, with this book, we are able to highlight the struggle that some people affected by dermatology endure then it will have been a worthwhile endeavour.

Carl Walker
Linda Papadopoulos
2004

Acknowledgments

We would like to thank our publishers and editors at Cambridge University Press, particularly Pauline Graham and Betty Fulford for their continued support, encouragement and feedback throughout the development of this book.

We have valued our contact with the Acne Support Group and the UK Vitiligo Society and particularly with Ms Maxine Whitton, a patient and professional whose inspirational spirit and priceless energy and commitment continue to directly and indirectly benefit psychodermatology patients the world over.

Finally, we would like to thank the patients and their families that have given their time to take part in our research over the years. In a field where it can be particularly difficult to expose themselves to the research process, their time, energy and bravery have allowed researchers and professionals alike to create a body of work which will help the population of skin disease patients as a whole.

Introduction

Carl Walker

'…You become introverted, avoid contact, become depressed, obsessive in looking at other people, hoping to see someone else who is affected. You undergo a personality change very slowly and bit by bit, a strong person is reduced to isolation. You become angry, sad and desperate. After time, it becomes an operation just to go out of your front door …'. 27-year-old female discussing her 15-year vitiligo history.

APGS Call for Evidence (2003)

The skin has long been recognised as the 'organ of expression' (Sack, 1928) and serves as the boundary between ourselves and the outside world, a 'first point of contact' when strangers meet us. It is also the largest organ of the body. The ways in which the skin can react to many different stimuli, both physiological (i.e. a rash caused by an external noxious substance) and psychological (an individual may blush when feeling embarrassed) highlight the complexity of the relationship between the skin, and external and internal factors. Dermatological disorders have an immediate impact on tactile communication, sexual contact and bodily interaction in particular and fear, anxiety and shame as well as sexual pleasure and excitement can be indicated visibly by growing pale, blushing and hair rising (Van Moffaert, 1992).

Unlike most internal illnesses, skin disease is often immediately visible to others and therefore people suffering from dermatological conditions may suffer social and emotional consequences. While disfigurement may have an impact on psychosocial functioning, relatively little attention has been paid to the psychosocial problems experienced by skin disease sufferers. Skin disease patients have direct access to their skin lesions and so can have a very direct impact on the progress of their condition and this is not the case with many other diseases. Since most skin conditions are accompanied by pain and discomfort, it can be difficult to assess the differential and combined effects of the physiological and psychosocial aspects of the condition on an individual's quality of life and self-esteem. However, psychological factors have long been known to be associated with dermatological conditions (Wilson, 1863; Engles, 1982) but only recently has there has been an accumulation of literature on the link between adult dermatology and psychosocial problems (e.g. Al'Abadie, 1994; Papadopoulos & Bor, 1999). Some of the issues which have been explored in recent research have tended to focus on morbidity in the areas of depression, anxiety, self-esteem, body image, quality of life and relationship/sexual issues (Papadopoulos & Walker, 2003). This focus on the potential psychosocial conflict caused by dermatological conditions indicates the range of issues pertinent to the holistic experience of skin disease.

Skin disease and psychology: a multitude of links

Psychological factors have been linked to dermatological illness in several and varied ways. Some authors have linked the aetiology of cutaneous illness to various psychological morbidities, ranging from Freud's conception of hysterical conversion mechanisms (Strachey, 2001) to Sheppard et al.'s (1986) notion of specific neurophysiological disturbances. Psychocutaneous phenomena have been classified in the past using personality-specific conflict and cutaneous symptoms (Obermeyer, 1985) and it was not until 1983 that Koblenzer posited a classification system comprising three specific, main categories of psychocutaneous illness:

- Conditions that are exclusively psychological in origin.
- Conditions in which strong psychogenic factors are implicated (i.e. urticaria).
- Conditions which are dependent on genetic and environmental factors but in which the course of the disease is substantially influenced by stress (vitiligo, eczema).

In 1992, Koblenzer modified this taxonomy to account for developments in the understanding of the influence of immune factors and the system became:

- Cutaneous manifestations of psychiatric disease.
- The effect of psychosocial stress on latent or a manifestation of cutaneous disease.
- The somatopsychic effect.

It has been estimated that between 40% and 80% of patients attending a dermatological outpatient clinic have experienced significant psychological or psychiatric problems, and Cotterill (1989) posited that these patients arose from five convenient and more detailed classifications:

- Individuals who experience psychosocial morbidity such as depression as a result of their skin disease. Visibility is considered to play a particular role in this group and it is not uncommon for these feelings to develop towards suicidal ideation.
- A more contentious group are those patients in whom it is believed that their skin disease has developed as a result of exposure to excessive stress or strain. Whilst this is a difficult area to quantify, there are considerable data (Van Moffaert, 1992;

Liu et al., 1996; Papadopoulos et al., 1998) to indicate that stress plays a profound role in the precipitation of a number of skin diseases including vitiligo, eczema, psoriasis, acne and urticaria.

- A third group of patients are those which present with factitious disorders such as dermatitis artefacta, trichotillomania, and oedema of the legs or arms.
- Some patients suffer dermatological delusional disease in which the commonest psychiatric assessment reveals depression. Patients present with some physical complaint relating to the skin or hair and delusions of parasitosis, the most common of these conditions is actually very rare. These patients are generally regarded to have monosymptomatic hypochondriacal psychosis.
- Finally, there is a group of patients who may develop dermatological disorders as a result of pharmaceutical therapy and the induction of acne and psoriasis in susceptible individuals who imbibe lithium is one example.

Skin diseases are more often than not accompanied by changes in the person's physical appearance and these changes are often obvious to others. This generates two major consequences. Firstly, the visibility of the condition may well be noticeable to others and draw people's attention. This can remove the feeling of personal control from the sufferer, as they no longer control when and how others know about their disease. It can often feel like their condition becomes 'public property' whereas many non-visible, internal diseases allow the sufferer to control who knows about their condition and when.

Secondly, skin disease has often been associated with myths surrounding lack of hygiene and contagion (Kleinman, 1988). This can influence others to act negatively towards the sufferer and hence often generate feelings of profound stigma. The fact that skin disease can often be progressive and episodic means that sufferers can sometimes feel that they constantly have to adapt to the changes in their physical appearance. It is often found that patients begin to feel handicapped and avoid social situations where their skin disease can be viewed by others and they can tend to have a poorer body image and lower self-esteem than the general population (Papadopoulos et al., 1999).

The episodic nature of many skin conditions also affects the way that patients conceptualise the cause of their condition. Uncertain aetiology combined with oscillating severity can cause sufferers to generate their own reasoning for their periods of exacerbation (Papadopoulos & Walker, 2003). This can lead to the avoidance of behaviours, places and events that may have no actual significance as regards symptom severity and this avoidance can be detrimental to the individual's quality of life. Negative reactions from others and a fear of such reactions can be one challenge of the skin disease experience that has to be met. The 'just world hypothesis', the idea that a person must somehow deserve their disfigurement as an appropriate punishment for previous transgressions (Goffman, 1968) together with the fear of contagion and uncertainty as to how to approach an individual with a visible difference can combine to make the experience of having a skin disease deeply challenging. Often, when people develop any severe or chronic ailment, they will question why they have developed the condition or what they have done to deserve this disease. This kind of thought process often implies a sense of punishment for some kind of wrongdoing and can carry feelings of guilt. Indeed, very often people with skin diseases link skin lesions to sexual causation and contagion themselves. Furthermore, when there is an insult to one's 'normal' sense of self which falls short of the 'ideal self', feelings of shame often ensue. Thoughts and concerns about the skin lesion are often displaced onto the self as a whole, as though patients form the syllogism: skin lesions are ugly, I have skin lesions, therefore I am ugly (Papadopoulos & Walker, 2003).

Updike (1990) has written eloquently about the enacted stigma of the psoriasis sufferer. He believed that the tendency for non-sufferers to turn away from people with skin disease or to feel disconcerted stems from a fleeting identification with the person who is afflicted. The affected person symbolises our own vulnerability and imperfection, our defensiveness and lack of autonomy. Updike speculates that we turn away from those who remind us of our own inherent humanity and vulnerability.

Skin disease and body image

To understand the social and psychological experience of living with a skin disease, it is essential for health professionals to understand patients' cognitions and the ways in which they represent their illness and their sense of self (Weinman et al., 2000).

Body image can be hypothesised as the 'inside view' that pertains to our own highly personalised experiences of our looks. For many people in society, body experiences are fraught with discontent, unhappiness and self-conscious preoccupation, and body image problems are difficulties in their own right, contributing as they do to a large range of psychological disturbances (Papadopoulos & Walker, 2003).

Early in the 20th century, body image concepts and studies had a tendency to focus on neurologically impaired patients. Although this brought the area of body image into the domain of scientific study, little attention was paid to the psychological aspects of body experience. More recently this has changed and in the past 20 years, much of the research on body image has emanated from a burgeoning interest in clinical eating disorders. Indeed much has been gained from this marriage of body image and eating disorders research but there have also been detrimental consequences (Cash & Brown, 1987). Body image has tended to become synonymous with either distorted body width estimates or a general emphasis on weight. As such, other aspects of body image such as skin disease have tended to be sidelined.

Cash and Pruzinsky (1990) delineated several integrative themes from the body image literature and concluded that body images were multifaceted and referred to perceptions, feelings and thoughts about the body. Body image feelings are intertwined with feelings about the self and body images have a strong social component. That is, interpersonal meaning and cultural socialisation define the social meaning of physical aesthetics and the personal meanings of an individual's physical characteristics. Furthermore, Cash and Pruzinsky showed that body images were not static but could operate on both trait and state levels, and so could be free to interact with the episodic nature of a range of factors including external, social events and the presence of a disfiguring condition such as skin disease. This is particularly relevant to skin disease patients since their conceptualisation of their body image may vary with the episodic nature and visibility of their disease (Thompson et al., 2002).

It has been reported that there are moderate associations between body dissatisfaction and poor psychological adjustment for men and women across the lifespan (Cash, 1985) and research has revealed that evaluative body image accounts for around a quarter to a third of variance in global self-esteem (Cash & Pruzinsky, 1990). As such, body satisfaction can have a considerable influence on psychosocial health. The literature has also shown a relationship between body satisfaction and depression (Noles et al., 1985), social confidence and social evaluation anxiety (Cash, 1993).

Self-schema(s) and body image

The core of body image dissatisfaction is a discrepancy between a person's perceived body and their ideal body. A failure to match these leads to self-criticism, guilt and low self-worth. Self-schema is a mental representation of those elements that make an individual different from other people. Myers and Biocca (1992) view a person's body image as one aspect of the mental representation that constitutes the self. As with other aspects of the self, the body image is a mental construction, not an objective evaluation. The authors believe that a number of reference points exist that a person will draw upon when constructing their mental model of body image. These include the 'socially represented ideal body' (ideals represented in the media, and drawn from peers and family), the objective body and the 'internalised ideal body' (a compromise between the objective body and the socially represented ideal). They argue that the body image is elastic in that its reference points frequently change since it depends on mood and the presence of social cues.

Cash and Pruzinsky (1990) believe that specific contextual events serve to activate schema-driven processing of information about, and self-appraisals of, one's body appearance. Implicit or internal dialogues such as automatic thoughts, interpretations and conclusions are termed 'private body talk'. In the case of individuals with skin disease who have a negative body image, this private talk can reflect habitual and faulty patterns of reasoning and the commission of specific cognitive errors. Among the defensive actions which may arise from these cognition's are avoidant and concealment behaviours, compulsive correcting rituals and social reassurance seeking.

The psychological impact of skin disease

It has been suggested that people whose appearance deviates from the norm have a more acute sense of awareness of their own bodies and the associated pressure to comply with social standards. This pressure has personal and social implications such as affecting relationships and hobbies (Porter et al., 1987), quality of life and expectations (Lanigan & Cotterill, 1989), and career aspirations (Goldberg et al., 1975).

Research into the manifestations of psychocutaneous disorders has led to an increasing awareness of the psychosocial effects associated with skin disease. These include depression, a decreased sense of body image and self-esteem, sexual and relationship difficulties, and a general reduction in quality of life (Dungey & Busselmeir, 1982; Obermeyer, 1985; Porter et al., 1987; Papadopoulos et al., 1999). Indeed, research has shown that people with skin disease experience higher levels of psychological and social distress (Root et al., 1994), poorer body image and lower self-esteem than the general population (Papadopoulos et al., 1999) and higher avoidance of situations where their skin may be exposed (Rubinow et al., 1987). Leary and colleagues (1998) suggest that the degree of social anxiety depends on a person's confidence regarding their ability to successfully manage the impression they make and it has been shown that social anxiety is a mediating factor between the severity of a disfiguring condition and an individual's emotional reactions.

An eclectic group of skin disease outpatients reported that their lives had been affected by skin disease in many ways (Jowett & Ryan, 1985). They reported difficulties in their relationships and poorer employment opportunities due to their skin disease, not to mention the damage that they felt their skin disease had afflicted on their self-esteem. Furthermore, functional and interpersonal problems in the workplace, increased anxiety and lack of confidence were also cited. Many patients feel that their sexual relationships and ability to find a partner have also suffered due to their skin condition (Porter et al., 1990). Furthermore, a British survey of acne patients showed unemployment levels in acne participants to be significantly higher than control participants (Cunliffe, 1986).

There is also evidence for cross-cultural stigmatisation due to skin disease. A striking example of this is the case of onchocercal skin disease (OSD), a disfiguring skin disease mostly found in Africa and associated with river blindness (onchocerciasis). Through a series of interviews with OSD sufferers in five different African sites, it was concluded that attitudes towards stigmatising illnesses showed strong similarity over the geographical and cultural areas specified in the study (Vlassoff et al., 2000).

Perhaps one of the crucial myths that permeates the lay discourse on skin disease is that of the severity of the condition being in some way related to a fixed psychosocial morbidity as experienced by the sufferer. This myth can help to form a barrier between the patient and friends, family and health professionals when outsiders automatically assume that a small or invisible lesion of dermatitis should not affect the psychological health of the sufferer. Thompson and Kent (2001) note that there is considerable evidence to suggest that self-perceived appearance, the view from the inside, is actually limited in its relationship with the social reality of appearance (Ben-Tovim & Walker, 1995; Robinson et al., 1996; Kleve et al., 2002).

Management

Psychosomatic management in dermatoses requires a perspective beyond the skin and its lesions. This means a more holistic perspective, with the use of anamnestic techniques and an adaptation of the physician/patient relationship. Many psychotherapeutic approaches, ranging from orthodox psychoanalysis to cognitive–behavioural therapy, biofeedback, behavioural conditioning and insight-orientated psychotherapy, have been employed in the treatment of dermatological disorders but the assessment of these psychological techniques in general has been inadequate (Van Moffaert, 1992). However, the incorporation of psychotherapeutic techniques into the domain of dermatology do generally improve patients' quality of life and at the least, do no harm. One of the principal problems with non-pharmacological treatments is that they lack the inherent appeal of drug studies to a scientific community. Drug studies allow the elucidation of chemical structures, physiological and biochemical processes, and so forth. Concrete constructs such as these allow definitive conclusions whereas non-pharmacological treatments allay a complexity of response that can be difficult to fully appreciate.

As mentioned, the series of changes that can affect individuals with visible medical conditions can be profound and there has been an increase in interest in the role of psychological therapy and visible medical issues in recent years. The practice of psychodermatology requires an eclectic approach and a monoform treatment of psychosomatic dermatosis is bound to be ineffective (Brown & Fromm, 1987). Problems that often exist in the current medical context is the lack of breadth in the knowledge of health professionals. General practitioners (GPs) often feel ill informed in the area of dermatology and dermatologists themselves can feel ill at ease with treatments that belong to the psychological field. However, the work that has addressed the application and efficacy of psychological interventions has shown that they appear to offer a useful adjunct to standard medical treatment.

Theoretical models and psychodermatology

Contextualing a review of any discipline requires that the discipline be placed within a theoretical and historical framework, and this approach is appropriate for psychodermatology. By the 1950s, the incidence of contagious diseases had declined rapidly and non-contagious diseases were on the increase. These included diseases that are related to lifestyle variables such as lung cancer and heart disease. Improved hygiene, vaccines and general medical treatment led to longer-life expectancy and the effects of health-compromising behaviours such as smoking, drinking, alcohol and poor diet had a growing effect on health. As a consequence of the limitations of the biomedical model and the change in disease statistics, researchers in the fields of health, psychology and medicine had begun to focus on the biopsychosocial model, a model that posits the fundamental assumption that health and illness are consequences of the interplay between psychological, biological and social factors (Engel, 1977). The biopsychosocial model maintains that health and illness are caused by multiple factors and produce multiple effects (Taylor, 1999). Interestingly, however, this perspective was not necessarily novel with respect to skin disease since a systemic view of the condition began to emerge as far back as the late 19th century with the work of dermatologists like Tuke (1884) and Beard (1880).

The diatheses–stress paradigm

Although we know that emotional factors can influence a wide range of medical conditions, we know less about why some people develop one disease in the presence of psychosocial stress while others develop no disease or a completely different set of symptoms. In order to understand this, it is necessary to understand the interaction between environmental and psychological variables in terms of an individual predisposition to a particular disorder. The diathesis–stress paradigm can sit as an adjunct to the biopsychosocial model (Meehl, 1962) and it focuses on the relationship between a predisposition to disease, the diathesis, and an environmental disturbance, the stress. With respect to skin disease, it has been suggested that sufferers inherit or gain a basic organ inferiority that will determine the results of psychological/biological upsets in such a way that autonomic activity may be directed towards the weak organ (Winchell & Watts, 1988). As regards dermatology, the weak organ is the skin.

Stress and dermatology

As far back as the 19th century, Hillier (1865), in working with eczema, implicated mental excitement, nervous debility and anxiety as the cause of these skin diseases. In 1982, Teshima and colleagues found that emotional stress had the capacity to influence the immune system to a great extent and that this would often manifest in cutaneous illness. They found that the tension in patients could lead to an enhancement of allergic reactions and these allergic patients were shown to improve with relaxation and autogenic training. There were also speculative implications for skin disease with the finding that the function of T-cells and the phagocytosis of macrophages were suppressed by induced stress. Furthermore, evidence of the strong relationship between the skin and the central nervous system (CNS) has been demonstrated by Ortonne and colleagues (1983) who noted that innervation of the CNS often produced blushing, perspiration and pallor.

Indeed, there has been considerable research that has investigated the role of emotional upsets antecedent to eruptions of skin disease with a number of conditions and consensus has suggested an association between stressful life events and the onset of skin conditions (Greismar, 1978; Invernizzi et al., 1988; Harper, 1992; Al'Abadie et al., 1994; Liu et al., 1996; Papadopoulos et al., 1998).

About the book

This book is intended to provide material of interest for a range of health professionals, including psychologists, psychiatrists, GPs, nurses and dermatologists as well as any other professionals who work with dermatology patients. Indeed this multidisciplinary readership is the key context behind the creation of the book. The book has been developed by academic psychologists, psychiatrists, psychotherapists and dermatologists, and it has taken the specific skills of each of these experienced professionals in order to provide the knowledge base behind the specific chapters. As health professionals involved with dermatology patients, it is our responsibility to be aware of all facets of skin disease and the way that these different facets interact to create the experience of suffering that can result from skin disease. Time constraints, financial restrictions and organisational inertia mean that this broadening of knowledge to better understand the physiological, psychological and social is not always possible. If anything, it is the purpose of this book to use the shared knowledge of our different contributing experts to help to broaden our perspective as health professionals both generally and specifically in the hope that skin disease patients receive a greater level of service in whatever health context they use.

In Chapter 2, Dr Leslie Millard, a Dermatologist from the University of Nottingham, discusses the multidisciplinary relationship between the physiological, psychological and social aspects of skin disease and the way that these factors can interact to influence the course of the disease is discussed. A treatment of recent research and approaches in the field of psychoneuroimmunology and how these relate to skin disease are discussed.

The psychiatric comorbidity in dermatological disorders is often one of the most important indices of the overall disability associated with these conditions and it is well established that significant psychiatric and psychosocial comorbidity is present in at least 30% of dermatology patients. Chapter 3 looks at the psychological morbidity associated with skin disease. Dr Madhulika Gupta, a Psychiatrist from the University of Ontario with expertise in the psychosocial aspects of skin disorder, highlights the relationship between dermatological disease and psychiatric comorbidity. This chapter focuses on the results of research on the relationship between skin disease and such psychosocial constructs as depression, suicidal ideation, social anxiety and body dysmorphic disorder.

In Chapter 4, Dr Gerry Kent from the University of Sheffield focuses on the stigma associated with disfigurement and skin disease particularly. Dr Kent, a Psychologist with a particular research interest in the stigma associated with vitiligo, highlights the myths and prejudice felt by those who are visibly different. By addressing the types of stigmatisation that people encounter, the content and effects of these experiences, the reasons why stigmatisation occurs and the ways in which we might reduce stigmatisation as well as a consideration of future research possibilities, Dr Kent comprehensively addresses the different ways in which people can feel stigmatised and the responses to this stigma.

Chapter 5 elaborates on factors that impact upon the adaptation and coping process. Dr Andrew Thompson, a Clinical Psychologist from the University of Sheffield who has published widely on the topic of skin disease and coping, discusses the various behavioural and cognitive changes that may accompany the onset of a skin condition. This chapter reviews the literature pertaining to adjusting to life with a chronic dermatological condition and details the factors that play key mediating roles in explaining individual variation in coping and adjustment.

The role and significance of intimate relationships in adjusting to skin disease is a neglected area in dermatology, despite evidence that partners are usually the most important source of support when facing ill health. Previous chapters have described the emotional and psychological effects of skin disease on the individual but skin disease often has an impact on relationships and Chapter 6 considers this impact and focuses on some of the relationship contexts in which difficulties regarding the skin condition may arise. Issues covered include the impact of skin disease on relationships, appearance and physical attraction, communication problems and sexuality. This chapter is contributed by Litsa Anthis from London

Metropolitan University, a counselling psychologist with extensive clinical and research experience working with skin disease patients around the world.

Since the psychological problems associated with a child's medical condition can have long-term implications, addressing these problems could be even more crucial for children than it is for adults. Although skin disease is very common among children and young people, there is surprisingly little research on the psychological impact of skin disease in childhood. Despite this lack of research, there is widespread acknowledgement of the impact of skin disease on the psychological well-being, and quality of life of children and their families. Chapter 7 addresses the key issues in understanding the relationship between skin disorders and psychological factors for children. It describes current theoretical models of the psychological impact of physical disease on children and their families as well as reviewing intervention strategies and methods of improving the psychological outcome for the children and their families. Dr Penny Titman, a Clinical Psychologist from Great Ormond Street Hospital for Children and an expert in the psychosocial aspects of paediatric dermatology, uses this chapter to discuss these distinct challenges to this population of skin disease patients.

On a practical level, dermatology deals with an organ that can be readily seen and touched. From intrusive questions to rude comments, relationship issues to depression, cutaneous conditions can have a devastating on the life of many sufferers. Chapter 8 will examine the use of counselling in addressing the issues faced by skin disease patients and will review the most frequently used psychological treatments. Their efficacy will be critically evaluated and recommendations for treatment will be made that take into account the potential challenges faced by people with skin problems. This chapter is contributed by Dr Linda Papadopoulos, a Reader in Psychology at London Metropolitan University and Co-editor of this book. Dr Papadopoulos uses her considerable research and clinical experience to highlight the potential benefits of psychotherapy to dermatology patients.

Research technique and methodology is crucial to any academic discipline and Chapter 9 will critically focus on the techniques and methodology used to assess quality of life and outcome in the health disciplines that comprise psychodermatology. Dr Andrew Finlay, a leading Dermatologist from the University of Wales College of Medicine and an expert in the psychometric issues prevalent in the field of psychodermatology makes recommendations for future directions.

Dr Carl Walker, Co-editor and a Health Psychologist from University College London with wide practical and research experience in psychodermatology, uses Chapter 10 to draw together the research findings to date within a theoretical framework that emphasises our understanding the importance of the beliefs people hold about their skin disease. Real-life anecdotal illustrations of the effect that skin disease can have on sufferers are provided in order to frame some of the aforementioned theory of earlier chapters within an everyday colloquial context. This chapter also discusses the issues facing psychodermatology as a multidiscipline and the role of psychodermatology in the future, emphasising the ways in which the implementation of psychological knowledge can benefit the health professionals that work with skin disease patients and how they can help the patients themselves.

REFERENCES

Al'Abadie, M.S.K., Kent, G.G., & Gawkrodger, D.J. (1994). The relationship between stress and the onset and exacerbation of psoriasis and other skin conditions. *British Journal of Dermatology*, **130**, 199–203.

The All Parliamentary Group on Skin (2003). *Call for Evidence*.

Beard, G.M. (1880). *What Constitutes a Discovery in Science?* New York.

Ben-Tovim, D.I., & Walker, M.K. (1995). Body image, disfigurement and disability. *Journal of Psychosomatic Research*, **39**(3), 283–291.

Brown, D.P., & Fromm, E. (1987). *Hypnosis and Behavioral Medicine*. Hillsdale, NJ: Erlbaum.

Cash, T.F. (1985). Physical appearance and mental health. In: J.A. Graham & A. Kligman (Eds), *Psychology of Cosmetic Treatments*. New York: Praeger Scientific.

Cash, T.F. (1993). Body-image attitudes among obese enrollees in a commercial weight-loss program. *Perceptual and Motor Skills*, **77**, 1099–1103.

Cash, T.F., & Brown, T.A. (1987). Body image in anorexia nervosa and bulimia nervosa: a review of the literature. *Behavior Modification*, **11**, 487–521.

Cash, T.F., & Pruzinsky, T. (1990). *Body Images: Development, Deviance and Change*. New York: Guildford Publications Inc.

Cotterill, J.A. (1989). Psychiatry and the skin. *British Journal of Hospital Medicine*, **42**, 401–404.

Cunliffe, W.J. (1986). Unemployment and acne. *British Journal of Dermatology*, **115**, 386.

Dungey, R.K., & Busselmeir, T.J. (1982). Medical and psychosocial aspects of psoriasis. *Health and Social Work*, **5**, 140–147.

Engel, G.L. (1977). The need for a new medical model: a challenge for biomedicine. *Science*, **196**, 129–136.

Engles, W.D. (1982). Dermatologic disorders. *Psychosomatics*, **23**, 1209–1219.

Goffman, E. (1968). *Stigma – Notes on the Management of Spoiled Identity*. Harmondsworth: Penguin Books.

Greismar, R.D. (1978). Emotionally triggered disease in dermatological practice. *Psychiatric Annals*, **8**, 49–56.

Goldberg, P., Bernstein, N., & Crosby, R. (1975). Vocational development of adolescents with burn injury. *Rehabilitation Counselling Bulletin*, **18**, 140–146.

Harper, J. (1992). Vitiligo: a questionnaire study. Unpublished research.

Hillier, T. (1865). *Handbook of Skin Disease*. London: Walton & Maberly.

Invernizzi, G., Gala, G., Bovio, L., Conte, G., Manca, G., Polenghi, M., & Russo, R. (1988). Onset of psoriasis: the role of life events. *Medical Science Research*, **16**, 143–144.

Jowett, S., & Ryan, T. (1985). Skin disease and handicap: an analysis of the impact of skin conditions. *Social Science and Medicine*, **20(4)**, 425–429.

Kleinman, A. (1988). *The Illness Narratives: Suffering, Healing, and the Human Condition*. New York: Basic Books, Inc.

Kleve, L., Rumsey, N., Wyn-Williams, M., & White, P. (2002). The effectiveness of cognitive–behavioural interventions provided at Outlook: a disfigurement support unit. *Journal of Evaluation in Clinical Practice*, **8(4)**, 387–395.

Koblenzer, C.S. (1992). Cutaneous manifestations of psychiatric disease that commonly present to the dermatologist – diagnoses and treatment. *International Journal of Psychiatry in Medicine*, **22(1)**, 47–63.

Koblenzer, C.S. (1983). Psychosomatic concepts in dermatology. A dermatologist–psychoanalyst's viewpoint. *Archives of Dermatology*, **119(6)**, 501–512.

Lanigan, S.W., & Cotterill, J.A. (1989). Psychological disabilities amongst patients with port-wine stain. *British Journal of Dermatology*, **121**, 209–215.

Leary, M.R., Rapp, S.R., Herbst, K.C., Exum, M.L., & Feldman, S.R. (1998). Interpersonal concerns and psychological difficulties of psoriasis patients: effects of disease severity and fear of negative evaluation. *Health Psychology*, **17**, 530–536.

Liu, P.Y., Bondesson, L., & Johansson, W.L.O. (1996). The occurrence of cutaneous nerve endings and neuropeptides in vitiligo vulgaris: a case control study. *Archives of Dermatology*, **288**, 670–675.

Meehl, P.E. (1962). Schizotaxia, schizotypy, schizophrenia. *American Psychologist*, **17**, 827–838.

Myers, P., & Biocca, F. (1992). The elastic body image: the effects of television advertising and programming on body image distortions in young women. *Journal of Communication*, **42**, 108–133.

Noles, S.W., Cash, T.F., & Winstead, B.A. (1985). Body image, physical attractiveness, and depression. *Journal of Consulting and Clinical Psychology*, **53**, 88–94.

Obermeyer, A. (1985). *Psychoses and Disorders of the Skin: Psychocutaneous Medicine*. Illinois: Thomas Publishing.

Ortonne, J.P. (1983). *Vitiligo and Other Hypomelanoses of Hair and Skin*. New York, Plenum Publishing.

Papadopoulos, L., & Bor, R. (1999). *Psychological Approaches to Dermatology*. BPS Books. Leicester, UK.

Papadopoulos, L., & Walker, C.J. (2003). *Understanding Skin Problems*. John Wiley & Sons Ltd. Chichester.

Papadopoulos, L., Bor, R., Legg, C., & Hawk, J.L.M. (1998). Impact of stressful life events on the onset of vitiligo in adults: preliminary evidence for a psychological dimension in aetiology. *Clinical and Experimental Dermatology*, **23(6)**, 243–248.

Papadopoulos, L., Bor, R., & Legg, C. (1999). Coping with the disfiguring effects of vitiligo: a preliminary investigation into the effects of cognitive–behavioural therapy. *British Journal of Medical Psychology*, **72(3)**, 385–396.

Porter, J.R., Beuf, A.H., Lerner, A., & Nordlund, J. (1987). Response to cosmetic disfigurement: patients with vitiligo. *Cutis*, **39**, 493–494.

Porter, J.R., Beuf, A.H., Lerner, A., & Nordlund, J. (1990). The effect of vitiligo on sexual relationships. *Journal of American Academy of Dermatology*, **22**, 221–222.

Robinson, E., Rumsey, N., & Partridge, J.P. (1996). An evaluation of the impact of social interaction skills training for facially disfigured people. *British Journal of Plastic Surgery*, **49**, 281–289.

Root, S., Kent, G., & Al-Abadie, M. (1994). The relationship between disease severity, disability and psychological distress in patients undergoing PUVA treatment. *Dermatology*, **189**, 234–237.

Rubinow, D.R., Peck, G.L., & Squillace, K.M. (1987). Reduced anxiety and depression in cystic acne patients after successful treatment with oral isotretinoin. *Journal of American Academy Dermatology*, **17(1)**, 25–32.

Sack, T. (1928). As cited in F.A. Whitlock. (1976). *Psychophysiological Aspects of Skin Disease*. London: WB Saunders Limited.

Sheppard, N.P., O'Loughlin, S., & Malone, J.P. (1986). Psychogenic skin disease: a review of 35 cases. *British Journal of Psychiatry*, **149**, 636–643.

Strachey, J. (2001). *The Complete Psychological Works of Sigmund Freud: 'A Case of Hysteria', 'Three Essays on Sexuality' and Other Works*. Vintage.

Taylor, S.E. (1999). *Health Psychology*. McGraw-Hill. New York.

Teshima, H., Kubo, C., & Kihara, H. (1982). Psychosomatic aspects of skin disease from the standpoint of immunology. *Psychotherapy Psychosomatics*, **37**, 165–175.

Thompson, A., & Kent, G. (2001). Adjusting to disfigurement: processes involved in dealing with being visibly different. *Clinical Psychology Review*, **21(5)**, 663–682.

Thompson, R.A., Kent, G., & Smith, J.A. (2002). Living with vitiligo: dealing with difference. *British Journal of Health Psychology*, **7**, 213–225.

Tuke, D. (1884). *Influence of the Mind upon the Body*. London: Churchill.

Updike, J. (1990). *Self consciousness Memoirs*. London: Penguin Books.

Van Moffaert, M. (1992). Psychodermatology: an overview. *Psychotherapy and Psychosomatics*, **58**, 125–136.

Vlassoff, C., Weiss, M., Ovuga, E.B.L., Eneanya, C., Titi Nwel, P., Sunday Babalola, S., Awedoba, A.K., Theophilus, B., Cofie, P., & Shetabi, P. (2000). Gender and the stigma or onchocercal skin disease in Africa. *Social Science & Medicine*, **50**, 1353–1368.

Weinman, J., Petrie, K.J., Sharpe, N., & Walker, S. (2000). Causal attributions in patients and spouses following first-time myocardial infarction and subsequent lifestyle changes. *British Journal of Health Psychology*, **5**, 263–273.

Wilson, A. (1863). As cited in F.A. Whitlock (1976). *Psychophysiological Aspects of Skin Disease*. London: WB Saunders Limited.

Winchell, S.A., & Watts, R.A. (1988). Relaxation therapies in the treatment of psoriasis and possible psychophysiologic mechanisms. *Journal of the American Academy of Dermatology*, **18**, 101–104.

2

Psychoneuroimmunology

Leslie Millard

Introduction

There is a colloquial folk belief that there is an influence of 'mind over matter' and that this can influence the onset, progression and resolution of disease. That is, that the state of mind can, to some extent, have a significant bearing not only upon how an illness is perceived but also on its severity and content. The concept of 'well-being' is common to all cultures and associated with declarations of 'life forces', 'vital life energies', chi in Chinese, ki in Japanese and prana in Sanskrit. In the presence of physical symptoms and disease, how is it that we may gain a further understanding of the curative value of 'talking therapies' and the physical effect that they have on recovery? Why do patients with depression suffer more physical illness? Is it related to immune suppression (Irwin, 2002) and how is this effect mediated?

This chapter will describe briefly the historical relationship between diseases of the skin and neuropsychiatry. In addition it will survey the anatomy of the structures in the brain, nerves and skin, which are all embryologically derived from the ectoderm. They show their origins from the neural plate where both the central nervous system (CNS) and peripheral nerves develop from the neural crest, as do the cutaneous structures, melanocytes and Merckel cells (Bernstern, 1983). The functional relationships between the brain and the immune system are reviewed, as is the linkage by the autonomic nervous system and the neuro-endocrine outflow via the hypothalamus and the pituitary gland. Communication between the immune system and the brain is bi-directional and probably largely mediated by chemical messengers called neuropeptides, released within nerves and also locally at tissue sites, in this case, the skin. This neuro-immuno-cutaneos-endocrine system (NICE) (Panconesi & Hautmann, 1996; Sullivan et al., 1998) seems to form part of an integrated system relating behaviour to neuroendocrine and immune function.

The skin has a critical immune function, employing a large number of cell populations in a coordinated manner to respond to both extrinsic and intrinsic challenge. The epidermal cells, keratinocytes, dendritic cells, such as Langerhans cells and melanocytes, function with dermal structures, such as macrophages, mast cells, leucocytes and dermal dendritic cells to provide this immune reaction. The mechanisms involved include the cell-signalling interactions provided by the glycoproteins, termed cytokines, which are produced by different cell types in all organs and tissues. In basic terms they are classified as interleukins (ILs), colony stimulating factors (CSFs), interferons (IFNs) and tumour necrosis factors (TNFs). When binding to specific receptor sites, cytokines may upregulate or downregulate the inflammatory, proliferative and immune reactions in target cells. Cytokines may also inhibit or stimulate the production of further cytokines in a cascade of activity. Furthermore, cytokines can fundamentally influence the direction of T lymphocyte helper (Th) subset differentiation into either Th1, cell-mediated immune reactions or Th2, humoral immune responses.

History

It may appear that the relationship between skin disease and psychological or neurotic influences has been established for many years (Whitlock, 1976). However, the apparent imaginative leap between skin and psyche in works by early writers (Cullen, 1784; Wilson, 1867) who describe nervous influences on skin function mean just that and not a later interpretation that this means a psychological component (Hunter & MacAlpine, 1963). The term neurosis retained its essential meaning of a disordered nerve function without a structural pathology until 100 years later when the prefix 'psycho' was added for nervous diseases caused psychologically.

This was the great era of Beard, Wier Mitchell, Charcot and Freud, where the rise of psychosexual interpretative writings about cutaneous disease set the agenda for the 20th century. Thus for example, an astute observation by Kaposi (1895) that 'neuroses of the skin are diseases which are occasioned by a change in function of the cutaneous nerves without demonstrable alteration in the skin' was skewed by the psychoanalytic beliefs of the day. He wrote of pruritis vulvae where 'the patients suffer from all the possible symptoms of hysteria and may even be nymphomaniacal'. The early developments of psychosomatic medicine, and with it dermatology, were characterised by this schism between the *neuro*, meaning neurological causation and the *psychoneuro*, meaning psychological and personality factors.

Whole fields of research into hysteria, personality types in dermatoses and psychoanalysis in individuals with skin disease dominated the literature until critical evaluation stressing the need for stringent appraisal led to a decline in interest in psychosomatic dermatology. Dermatology had moved from a highly skilled, descriptive, clinical specialty with unsubstantiable theories of aetiology to an era of scientific questioning, skin pathology and biochemistry.

Studies of the physiology of itching, skin temperature and blood flow (Cormia & Kaykendall, 1953) under stress, as well as allergic responses after hypnosis (Black, 1969) reopened scientific enquiry and instigated a new impetus.

In 1964, Solomon and Moss introduced the term psychoimmunology in the paper 'Emotions, immunity, and disease: a speculative theoretical integration' but the real expansion of psychoneuroimmunology did not begin until the demonstration of behaviourally conditioned immunosupression by Adler and Cohen in 1975.

Initial studies of immune function in psychiatric patients had shown reduced lymphocyte numbers and diurnal variability in psychosis (Freeman & Elmadjian, 1947), and poorer antibody response to pertussis vaccination in schizophrenia. Further changes were shown in cellular immunocompetency and urinary stress cortisol levels in psychiatric patients (Kiecolt Glaser et al., 1984).

The clinical links between psychosomatic factors and skin disease is amply demonstrated by the fluctuations of remission and relapse which are seen in dermatological disorders as a result of stress and psychological events in patients' lives (Wang et al., 1990). There is a substantial body of evidence detailing the neural innervation of the skin with nerve fibres extending from the sub-cuticular tissue through the dermis and into the epidermis (Richards et al., 2001). The contact between nerve cells and epidermal cells was first recorded by Langerhans and Merckel whose names were appended to the cells. The former is a dendritic cell whose processes make contact with epidermal cell borders whilst the latter is an epidermal neuroendocrine structure in contact with nerve endings. Furthermore, ultrastructural studies have shown connections between keratinocytes, melanocytes and cutaneous mast cells at all levels in the skin (Hilliger et al., 1995).

Afferent pathway

The afferent neural anatomical pathway is well-known. Sensory perception is mediated by afferent sensory fibres beginning with peripheral sensory bodies specifically recording pain, pressure and temperature, such as Meissner's corpuscle, Pacinian corpuscles and free nerve endings. These sensations are relayed along the ascending spinal sensory pathways via myelinated A fibres and unmyelinated C fibres or cranial nerves to the thalamus in the cerebral cortex.

At this stage it is important to mention the vital function of some of these unmyelinated C afferent fibres, which also serve to secrete neuropeptides as an *efferent* function. These neuropeptides are a diverse group of peptides and amino acids (often fewer than 40 amino acids in length) which act as intercellular messengers either alone or in conjunction with others to effect neuroendocrine and immune actions in response to acute or chronic stimuli (Panconesi & Hautmann, 1996).

Efferent pathway

The functional response, that is the degree to which the stimulus is recognised as a stress, is determined by the individual perceptions of the magnitude and importance of the challenge. The degree of the effector response is determined by factors, which may suppress or magnify this reaction. Thus patient reactions to a bee sting can be demonstrably different. In the truly venom-allergic patient this may lead to an immediate dramatic immune-mediated anaphylaxis. Secondly, in the bee-phobic individual, fear and pain lead to autonomic vaso-vagal collapse because of a highly psychologically reactive drive. For most people who are stung there is recognition of the pain and a local inflammatory and immune reaction in the skin but no threat to general well-being. The bee-keeper may pay no attention at all to yet another sting because it is perceived as normal or suppressed possibly by an anergic mechanism and therefore not perceived as a threat.

Responses

Seyle (1946) proposed that organisms have the ability to adapt to acute changes in their status, for example the 'fight or flight' response in acute noxious injury. However with chronicity, such as repeated assaults, this may be replaced by anger and fear. Ultimately this can lead to a state of learned helplessness and chronic anxiety. However, reaction patterns cannot be generalised and Mason (1968) showed that steroid reactions to stress differed not only with types of stress but also with species.

Personality characteristics and coping styles have been related to immune responses to stress. Skin reactivity to allergens and predisposition to allergic disorders was weaker in individuals classified as passive, negative, anxious and impulsive (Jacobs et al., 1966; Freeman et al., 1967). Army recruits who were highly motivated but poorly performing were more susceptible to infectious mononucleosis (Kasl, 1979) and furthermore, Esterling (1990) found that students with repressive coping styles had higher Epstein–Barr Virus (EBV) titres, suggesting a reduction in memory T-cell responses to the virus. Support for this view was found in the work of Janner et al. (1988) who showed lower monocyte counts, higher eosinophil numbers and self-reported drug reactions in medical out-patients with similar coping styles. An appraisal of stress and skin disease is reviewed fully in Picardi and Abeni (2001).

To summarise, stressful influences initiating autonomic, neuroendocrine or immune responses are listed in Table 2.1.

Common stressful events appear to induce immune changes. Thus examination stress has been shown to delay immune reactivity to hepatitis vaccination and

Table 2.1. Stress producing stimuli

Psychogenic
Fear, rage, anger, frustration and helplessness

Environmental
Heat or cold, noise, pollutants, change in diurnal rhythms

Behavioural
Isolation, overcrowding, physical restraint, enforced starvation,
change in diet and hierarchical challenge

delay experimental wound healing (Marucha et al., 1998). Hernia surgery patients with high life stresses had lower lymphocyte responses to challenge before surgery and increased post-operative complications and longer lengths of stay (Linn et al., 1988).

Long-term stress may produce chronic immune dysfunction and the susceptibility to common cold and other upper respiratory viruses is increased in those with work 'burnout', job strain, unemployment and refugee status (Glaser et al., 2000; Sabioncello et al., 2000). These latter effects appear to involve the neuro-immuno-endocrine pathway.

The neuroendocrine pathway

Whatever the recognised stressor, the response is to trigger the neuroendocrine pathway via the hypothalamic–pituitary–adrenal (HPA) axis (Chrousos, 1995). The hypothalamic paraventricular nuclei stimulate the secretion of corticotrophin releasing hormone (CRH) and in addition, vasopressin. These travel down the hypophyseal-pituitary portal system to the anterior pituitary and release adreno-corticotropic hormone (ACTH). The adrenal cortex responds by secreting cortisone into the circulation and this classic feedback mechanism then suppresses ACTH, CRH and vasopressin.

During the neuroendocrine response, the autoimmune nervous system is also activated by the brainstem nuclei, predominantly the nucleus ceruleus, which provokes the production of noradrenaline and neuropeptides from spinal ganglia and the adrenal medulla. In addition, these neuropeptides released by autonomic stress systems, such as proopiomelanocortin exert a modulating control on both CRH-secreting neurons and pain control secretions in the hindbrain (Scholzen et al., 1998).

The neuromediators and neurohormones involved are predominantly neuropeptides, existing as small, simple compounds of 40 or less amino acids. The major group of neuropeptides include substance P (SP), calcitonin gene-related peptide (CGRP) and vasoactive intestinal peptide (VIP). Other significant neuropeptides

Table 2.2. Neuropeptides and their effect on skin cell type

Target cells	Neuropeptide		
	SP	CGRP	VIP
Endothelial	Proliferation permeability	Proliferation IL-8 secretion	Proliferation
Keratinocyte	Stimulate IL-1 and IL-8, Comitogen, LTB4, CGRP	Proliferation in conjunction with SP	Mitogenic proliferation
Lymphocyte	Proliferation IL-2 synthesis, B-cell differentiation	Chemotactic to T-cells, increases proliferation	NK cell activity
Macrophage	IL-1 and IL-6 synthesis	Impairs antigen presentation	
Mast cell	Histamine and TNF alpha release	Histamine and TNF alpha release	Histamine release
Monocyte	Chemotaxis, phagocytosis		Enhanced migration
Neutrophil	Chemotaxis, phagocytosis	Enhances chemotaxis	

are neuropeptide Y, somatostatin, neurokins A and B and the opiomelanocortins, which include the endorphins. More details can be found in Panconesi and Hautmann (1996) and Scholzen et al. (1998).

A brief summary of actions of important neuropeptides and their target cells is illustrated in Table 2.2. Cytokine responses are also indicated. There are fuller descriptions further on for specific skin diseases.

Changes in disease

The neuroendocrine effects of acute and chronic illness relate to the immediate 'fight or flight' reaction and chronic adaptation responses referred to above. Whereas the reactions occurring with chronicity tend to promote a predominantly immunosuppressive response, the acute feedback is now believed to consist of immune-enhancement consistent with an immediate survival mechanism (Sternberg, 2001).

The chronic immune response to stress is best recognised as an *immunosuppressive* reaction. It is thought to be mediated by provoking a change in T-helper cell response from Th1 whose main function is to promote cell-mediated immunity to Th2 cells which have a predominantly humoral immune function. Corticosteroids, via the HPA axis, induce the secretion of the cytokine IL-10, a key stage in the Th2 response, as well as suppressing IL-12, a cytokine essential for the induction of the Th1 response and suppression of Th2. This effect inhibits IL-12 expression by T cytotoxic and natural killer (NK) cells and inflammatory cytokines, such as IFN gamma.

The catecholamines released in chronic stress appear to have a related effect by inhibiting IL-12 and enhancing IL-10 (Hazko et al., 1998). Paradoxically it has been proposed that the acute stress reaction seen in inflammatory dermatoses, such as psoriasis and eczema, (Dhabar et al., 1996) is induced also by corticosteroids and catecholamines, which have a particular effect in the acute stress response of inducing enhanced cell-mediated immunity via INF gamma and the cytokine IL-2.

Animal studies (Jafarian-Tehrani & Sternberg, 1999) have suggested that the HPA axis response to stress may also be impaired in chronic stress, allowing a susceptibility to autoimmune diseases to emerge. The mechanism is unclear but similar observations in patients with atopic eczema (Buske-Kirschbaum et al., 1997) and rheumatoid disease (Gutierrez et al., 1999) have been recorded.

Cytokines in depression and anxiety

There is mounting evidence that both depression and depressive symptoms can induce immune dysregulation by the production of proinflammatory cytokines including IL-6 (Maes et al., 1998). Similar responses in chronic anxiety with the production of IL-6 and reduced IL-2 receptor production (which is an essential cytokine to counter infection) was deemed a factor in increased URTI episodes (Ravindran, 1995). Persistent elevation of pro-inflammatory cytokines may lead to chronicity in disease, poor healing and increased disability (Leventhal et al., 1998). It seems, therefore, that negative emotions can directly affect the immune system to up or down regulate the response via inflammatory cytokines. This affects not only immediate reaction to the challenge of infection, but also the mechanisms of inflammatory disease.

Inflammatory skin disease

The psychocutaneous responses in the commonest inflammatory dermatoses, namely atopic eczema and psoriasis, have been investigated at length and, in conjunction with cutaneous viral infections, are discussed in order to illustrate the complex interactions that can be involved in skin disease (Buske-Kirschbaum et al., 2001; Fortune et al., 2002). Atopic eczema is considered primarily a Th-2 mediated disease whilst psoriasis has mechanisms mediated by Th-1 pathways.

Atopic eczema

The psychosocial stressors implicated in atopic dermatitis are summarised in Table 2.3.

Table 2.3. Psychosocial stress in atopic eczema

Itching
Sleep disturbance
Withdrawal of touching
'allergic object relationship'
Diet modification stresses
Disfigurement reactions, such as rejection, secrecy
　　and aggression
Underachievement
Psychosexual difficulties
Parental distress

The influence of these factors, with regard to physical atopic disease, depends on both generic and specific individual features. Genetic factors play a significant role in the type and quality of response and the genes responsible for cytokines are being delineated (Leung, 2000).

Atopic dermatitis has been considered a prime example of a Th2 disease mechanism. In atopic dermatitis the presentation of immunoglobulin E (IgE) antigen appears to be one of the fundamental mechanisms intrinsic to the disease. IgE-allergen complex presentation by cutaneous Langerhans cells to circulating and tissue T-cells continue the response, which, in atopy, consists mainly of Th2 cells. There is an increased ratio of Th2 to Th1 cells in atopy leading to the increase in humoral immunity via cytokine IL-4. This induces IgE-producing B-cells and enhanced eosinophil activity via cytokine IL-5 (Leung, 2000; Blauvelt et al., 2003). The induction and maintainance of eosinophils in atopic skin is maintained by Th2 cytokines. These are instrumental in the production of additional chemokines which play a further role in recruiting immune cells to skin. These include eotaxin, Thymus and Activation Related Chemokine (TARC) and Regulated on Activation, T-cell Expressed and Secreted (RANTES). The degranulation of mast cells produces histamine which has local inflammatory and vasoactive effects on the skin. In addition, the direct effect of the neuro immunocutaneous system via the C-fibres stimulate the release of neuropeptides SP, CGRP, VIP and neurogenic factor (NGF). As listed in Table 2.1, these induce proliferative responses in leucocytes, monocytes, keratinocytes and importantly, mast cells. Cytokine release promotes further Th2 response, notably IL-10, a potent immunosuppressor of Th1 helper cells. Increased numbers of mast cells have been found in chronic atopic dermatitis (Singh et al., 1999). The catecholamines secreted after stress act in atopic eczema via beta adrenoreceptors on cells which stimulate intracellular phosphodiesterases to degrade cAMP and produce the cytokines IL-4 and IL-13 (Hanifin & Chan, 1999).

Therapeutic interventions within the complex NICE mechanisms promoting psychotherapeutic treatments have been reviewed (Buske-Kirschbaum, 2001; Gieler et al., 2003). Many of the psychotherapies are behaviour modification programmes directed towards itch-scratch relief. However, more broadly based psychotherapies were rated by patients as being as effective as topical steroids (Linner & Jemmee, 2001).

Psoriasis

Psoriasis, like atopic eczema, is an inflammatory skin disease with a multifactorial aetiology. It is a chronic, immune-mediated disorder (Kreuger, 1989) associated with significant physical and psychological morbidity. The psychological factors have been summarised by Ginsburg and Link (1989) and instruments have been developed to measure psoriasis-related stress (Wang et al., 1990; Fortune et al., 2002).

In psoriasis there is an overexpression of INF gamma and TNF alpha and a relative underexpression of the Th2 cytokines, IL-4 and IL-10. It appears that the T-cells involved are Th1 lymphocytes and that the disease may be influenced by a cell-mediated autoimmune process.

There is an early influx of T-cells into psoriatic lesions, increased antigen presentation in psoriatic cells and ablative effect with anti-T cell therapy, and the common antigens considered in the pathogenesis of psoriasis are bacterial proteins and superantigens.

However, clinical and histological features in psoriasis show the Koebner phenomenon on trauma, clearance of psoriatic plaque after desensitising injury, symmetry of clinical lesions and increased nerve density in psoriatic plaques, which have led to the proposal of a neurogenic hypothesis for the disease (Raychaudhuri et al., 1995; Raychaudhuri & Farber, 2000).

Nerve growth factor (NGF) is a peptide whose functions have been shown to stimulate and direct nerve growth. At a cellular level in skin it is mitogenic for keratinocytes and promotes the migration and degranulation of mast cells leading to dilated vessels and oedema. In addition to this promotion of the release of inflammatory mediators via mast cells, NGF also induces keratinocytes to produce the cytokine RANTES, a key participant in the activation of memory T-cells in psoriasis (Raychaudhuri & Farber, 2000). NGF, together with neuropeptides, have been shown to produce neutrophil response in psoriasis via CGRP and IL-8. They are mitogenic for keratinocytes and inhibitors of apoptosis (cell death) via SP, CGRP and VIP, and thus probably contribute to the influences producing the epidermal proliferation in psoriasis (Pincelli et al., 1997).

These sophisticated measurements in cutaneous biology are not matched by clinical correlations during non-pharmacological interventions in skin disease.

However, it was shown that a structured programme in the management of psychological distress with cognitive–behaviour management reduced relapse of disease. Furthermore, psychological distress impairs the clearance of psoriasis treated with photochemotherapy (Fortune et al., 2002). This is indirect evidence that these putative stress mechanisms have clinical importance.

Cutaneous viral infections

Patients with recurrent oro-facial herpes simplex virus (HSV) frequently relate this to a psychostressful event. The nature of the HSV is such that active infection occurs with the loss of antiviral control. The HSV is latent within the sensory dorsal root ganglion until some stimulus precipitates an activation where the virus migrates down the sensory nerves to the skin. The stimulae can be as variable as fever, trauma, infection and stress. Studies in recurrent HSV (Biondi & Zannino, 1997) show that there is a shift from the Th1-mediated T-cell control to a more primitive Th2 humoral response. Essential in this mechanism is the neuroendocrine stimulus to HPA corticosteroid secretion. This was found to produce an HSV IgE response and a poor cell-mediated immunity to the virus. The humoral response allows reactivation of active virus whereas T-cell type 2 responses are essential for virus killing.

Research into the relationship between life stress and human papillomavirus (HPV) and human immunodeficiency virus (HIV) suggests that major psychosocial events are implicated in immune decrements in HPV infections and tendency to intraepithelial neoplasia (Pereira et al., 2003). Further studies on the stress management effects on psychological, endocrinological and immune functioning in men with HIV infection suggested that psychotherapy had measureable beneficial effects. A 10-week, group-based cognitive–behavioural stress-management intervention showed reductions in catecholamine urine output, urine cortisol output and beneficial changes in CD8 cytotoxic and CD4 lymphocytes (Hickie et al., 1999).

Multifaceted cognitive–behavioural stress management reduced EBV capsid antigen and human herpesvirus: six antibody titres in HIV-seropositive men compared to controls. This reduction was thought to be as a result of a more stable cellular immune system not suppressed by inflammatory cytokines.

Conclusion

There is now a large body of evidence to conclude that immune modulation by psychosocial stressors or intervention can lead to health changes. There is an impressive spectrum of diseases, which seem to be influenced by proinflammatory cytokines. These can be directly stimulated by negative emotions and stressful experiences and indirectly stimulated by chronic or recurring infections.

There are many other dermatoses with a putative psychosomatic component, such as urticaria, alopecia areata and other psychological effects upon skin, like delayed wound healing (Augustin & Maier, 2003) requiring further investigation. The pathways of stress-skin interaction are becoming clearer and with them a further recognition that the clinical beliefs long held by dermatologists and psychologists, that stress influences disease, are being supported by objective immune measurement. However, easy clinical monitoring of the effects of psychological intervention upon the immune system with markers, such as levels of a cytokine (i.e. IL-6) are still propositions rather than practicalities. The value of psychological therapies in dermatological medicine is not in doubt although, as in the past, the establishment of measureable immune responses in tandem with clinical improvement to psychological therapies should convert more of the sceptics.

REFERENCES

Adler, R., & Cohen, N. (1975). Behaviourly conditioned immunosuppression. *Psychosomatic Medicine*, **37**, 333–340.

Augustin, M., & Maier, K. (2003). Psychosomatic aspects of chronic wounds. *Dermatology and Psychosomatics*, **4**, 5–13.

Bernstern, J.E. (1983). Neuropeptides and the skin. In: L.E. Goldsmith (Ed.), *Biochemistry and Physiology of the Skin*, New York: Oxford University Press, pp. 1217–1233.

Biondi, M., & Zannino, L.G. (1997). Psychological stress, neuroimmunomodulation and susceptibility to infectious diseases in animals and man: a review. *Psychotherapy and Psychosomatics*, **66**, 3–26.

Black, S. (1969). *Mind and Body*. London: Kimber, pp. 234–238.

Blauvelt, A., Hwang, S.T., & Udey, M.C. (2003). Allergic and immunologic diseases of the skin. *Journal of Allergy and Clinical Immunology*, **111(Suppl.)**, S560–S570.

Buske-Kirschbaum, A., Geiber, A., & Hellhammer, D. (2001). Psychobiological aspects of atopic dermatitis: an overview. *Psychotherapy and Psychosomatics*, **20**, 6–16.

Buske-Kirschbaum, A., Jobst, S., & Psycho, D., et al. (1997). Attenuated free cortual response to psychosocial stress in children with atopic dermatitis. *Psychosomatic Medicine*, **59**, 419–426.

Chrousos, G.O. (1995). The hypothalamus pituitary adrenal axis and immune-mediated inflammation. *New England Journal of Medicine*, **332**, 1351–1362.

Cormia, F.E., & Kaykendall, V. (1953). Experimental histamine pruritus: physical and environmental factors influencing development and severity. *Journal of Investigative Dermatology*, **20**, 429–436.

Cullen, W. (1784). *First Lives of the Practice of Physic*, 4th edn. Edinburgh: Elliot.

Dhabar, F.S., Miller, A.H., & McEwen, B.S. (1996). Stress induced changes in blood leucocyte distribution. Role of adrenal steroid hormones. *Journal of Immunology*, **157**, 1038–1044.

Esterling, B., Antoni, M., Kumar, M., & Scneiderman, N. (1990). Emotional repression, stress disclosure responses, and Epstein–Barr viral capsid antigen titres. *Psychosomatic Medicine*, **52**, 397–410.

Fortune, D.C., Richards, H.C., Griffith, C.E., & Main, C.J. (2002). Psychological stress, distress and disability in patients with psoriasis. *British Journal of Clinical Psychology*, **2**, 157–174.

Freeman, H., & Elmadjian, F. (1947). The relationship between blood sugar and lymphocyte levels in normal and psychotic patients. *Psychosomatic Medicine*, **9**, 226–233.

Freeman, E.H., Gorman, F.J., Singer, M.T., & Affelder, M.T. (1967). Personality variables and allergic skin reactivity: a cross validation study. *Psychosomatic Medicine*, **29**, 312–322.

Gieler, U., Niemeler, V., Kupefer, J., & Brosig, B. (2003). Psycho physiological aspects of atopic dermatitis. In: J. Koo, & C.S. Lee (Ed.), *Psychocutaneous Medicine*, New York: Dekker, pp. 108–114.

Ginsburg, I.H., & Link, B.C. (1989). Feelings of stigmatisation in psoriasis. *Journal of American Academic Dermatology*, **20**, 53–63.

Glaser, R., Sheridan, J.F., & Malarkey, W.B. (2000). Chronic stress modulates the immune response to a pneumococcal vaccine. *Psychosomatic Medicine*, **62**, 804–807.

Gutierrez, M.A., Garcia, M.E., & Rodriguez, J.A., et al. (1999). HPA axis function in patient with acute rheumatoid arthritis. *Journal of Rhematocology*, **26**, 2777–2781.

Hanifin, J., & Chan, S. (1999). Biochemical and immunological mechanisms in atopic dermatitis: new targets for emerging therapies. *Journal of American Academic Dermatology*, **41**, 72–77.

Hazko, G., Szabo, C., & Nemeth, Z.H., et al. (1998). Stimulation of beta-adrenoreceptors inhibit endotoxin induced IL-12 production in normal and IL-10 deficient mice. *Journal of Neuroimmunology*, **88**, 57–61.

Hickie, I., Bennett, B., Lloyd, A., Heath, A., & Martin, W. (1999). Complex genetic and environmental relationships between psychological distress, fatigue and immune functioning. *Psychology of Medicine*, **29**, 269–277.

Hilliger, M., Wang, L., & Johansson, D. (1995). Ultra structure evidence of nerve fibres within all vital layers of the human epidermis. *Journal of Investigative Dermatology*, **104**, 134–137.

Hunter, R., & MacAlpine, I. (1963). *Three Hundred Years of Psychiatry*, London: Oxford University Press.

Irwin, M. (2002). Psycho neuroimmunity of depression: clinical implications. *Brain Behaviour and Immunity*, **16**, 1–16.

Jacobs, M.A., Friedman, M.A., Franklin, M.J., & Anderson, L.S. (1966). Incidence of psychosomatic predisposing factors in allergic disorders. *Psychosomatic Medicine*, **28**, 679–695.

Jafarian-Tehrani, M., & Sternberg, G.M. (1999). Animal models of neuroimmune interactions in inflammatory diseases. *Journal of Neuroimmunology*, **100**, 13–20.

Janner, L.D., Swartz, G.E., & Leigh, H. (1988). The relationship between repressive and defensive coping styles and monocyte, eosinophil, and serum glucose levels. *Psychosomatic Medicine*, **50**, 567–575.

Kaposi, M. (1895). *Pathology and Treatment of the Skin*, New York: William Ward.

Kasl, S.V., Evans, A.S., & Neiderman, P.C. (1979). Psychosocial factors in the development of infectious mononucleosis. *Psychosomatic Medicine*, **41**, 445–466.

Kiecolt-Glaser, J.K., Ricker, D., George, J., Messick, G., Speicher, C.E., Garner, W., & Glaser, R. (1984). Urinary cortisol levels, cellular immunocompetency, and loneliness in psychiatric inpatients. *Psychosomatic Medicine*, **46**, 15–24.

Kreuger, J.G. (1989). The immune basis for the treatment of psoriasis with new biologic agents. *Journal of American Academic Dermatology*, **46**, 1–23.

Leventhal, H., Patrick, L., Leventhal, E.A., & Burns, E.A. (1998). Does stress emotion cause illness in elderly people. In: K.W. Schiae, & M.P. Lawton (Eds), *Annual Review of Gerontology and Geriatrics, Vol. 17 Focus on Emotion and Adult Development*. New York: Springer Publishing, pp. 138–84.

Leung, D.Y. (2000). Atopic dermatitis: new insights and opportunities for therapeutic intervention. *Journal of Allergy and Clinical Immunology*, **105**, 860–876.

Linn, B.S., Linn, M.W., & Klimas, N.G. (1988). Effects of psychophysical stress on surgical outcome. *Psychosomatic Medicine*, **50**, 230–244.

Linner, J., & Jemmee, G.B. (2001). Anxiety level and severity of skin condition and outcome of psychotherapy. *International Journal of Dermatology*, **40**, 632–636.

Maes, M., Lin, A., Delmeire, L., & Bosmans, E. (1998). The effects of psychological stress on humans: increased productivity of pro-inflammatory cytokines and Th-1 like response in stress induced anxiety. *Cytokine*, **10**, 313–318.

Marucha, P.T., Keicolt-Glaser, J.K., & Favagehi, M. (1998). Mucosal wound healing is impaired by examination stress. *Psychosomatic Medicine*, **60**, 362–365.

Mason, J.W. (1968). Over-all normal balance as a key to endocrine function. *Psychosomatic Medicine*, **20**, 791–808.

Panconesi, E., & Hautmann, C. (1996). Pathophysiology of stress in dermatology. *Dermatologic Clinics*, **14**, 319–341.

Pereira, D.B., Antoni, M.H., & Danielson, A., et al. (2003). Life stress and cervical squamous intraepithelial lesion in woman with HPV and HIV. *Psychosomatic Medicine*, **65**, 427–434.

Picardi, A., & Abeni, D. (2001). Stressful life events and skin disease: disentangling evidence from myth. *Psychotherapy and Psychosomtics*, **70**, 118–136.

Pincelli, C., Haake, A.R., & Benassi, L., et al. (1997). Autocrine nerve growth factor protects human keratinocytes from apoptosis. *Journal of Investigative Dermatology*, **109**, 751–764.

Raychaudhuri, S.P., & Farber, E.M. (2000). Neuroimmunologic aspects of psoriasis. *Cutis*, **68**, 357–363.

Raychaudhuri, S.P., Rein, G., & Farber, E.M. (1995). Neuropathogenesis and neuropharmacology of psoriasis. *International Journal of Dermatology*, **34**, 685–693.

Richards, H., Fortune, D.G., & Griffiths, C.E.M. (2001). The contribution of perceptions of stigmatisation to disability in patients with psoriasis. *Journal of Psychosomatic Research*, **50**, 11–15.

Ravindran, A.V., Griffiths, J., Merali, Z., & Anisman, H. (1995). Lymphocyte subsets associated with major depression and dysthymia. *Psychosomatic Medicine*, **57**, 555–563.

Sabioncello, A., Rabatic, S., Tomasic, J., & Dekaris, D. (2000). Immune, endocrine and psychological responses in civilians displaced by war. *Psychosomatic Medicine*, **62**, 502–508.

Seyle, H. (1946). The general adaptive syndrome and diseases of adaptation. *Journal of Clinical Endocrinology*, **6**, 117–230.

Scholzen, T., Armstrong, C.A., & Bunnett, N.W. (1998). Neuropeptides in the skin: interactions between the neuroendocrine and the skin immune system. *Experimental Dermatology*, **7**, 81–96.

Singh, L., Pang, X., & Alexacos, N., et al. (1999). Acute immobilisation stress triggers skin mast cell degranulation via corticotrophin-releasing hormone, neurotensin and substance P: A link to neurogenic skin disorders. *Brain Behaviour Immunology*, **13**, 225–239.

Solomon, G.F., & Moss, R.H. (1964). Emotions, immunity and disease; a speculative theoretical integration. *Archives of General Psychiatry*, **11**, 657–674.

Sternberg, G.M. (2001). Neuroendocrine regulation of autoimmune/inflammatory disease. *Journal of Endocrinology*, **169**, 425–435.

Sullivan, R.L., Lipper, G., & Lerner, E.A. (1998). The neuro-immuno-cutaneous endocrine network; relationship of mind and skin. *Archives of Dermotology*, **134**, 1431–1435.

Wang, L., Hillinger, M., & Jernberj, T., et al. (1990). Protein gene product 0.5. Immunoreactive nerve tissues and cells in human skin. *Cell Tissue Research*, **261**, 25–33.

Whitlock, F.A. (1976). *Psycho physiological aspects of skin disease*. London, WB Sanderson, pp. 1–13.

Wilson, E. (1867). *Diseases of the skin*. London, Churchill.

3

Psychiatric comorbidity in dermatological disorders

Madhulika A. Gupta

Introduction

The psychiatric comorbidity in dermatological disorders is often one of the most important indices of the overall disability associated with the dermatological condition (Panconesi, 1984; Gupta & Gupta, 1996; Woodruff et al., 1997; Picardi et al., 2000; Gupta & Gupta, 2003; Picardi et al., 2004; Sampogna et al., 2004). It is well established that significant psychiatric and psychosocial comorbidity is present in at least 30% of dermatological patients, and untreated comorbid psychiatric disorders may adversely affect the response of the dermatological disorder to standard dermatological therapies (Picardi et al., 2003). Psychiatric pathology is important in both (i) the cutaneous associations of primary psychiatric disorders such as delusional states and some of the self-inflicted dermatoses such as dermatitis artefacta, and (ii) a wide range of primary dermatological disorders that have psychiatric comorbidity. Any dermatological disorder that is cosmetically disfiguring can be associated with significant psychiatric morbidity. Stress-related neuroimmunomodulation may affect the course of viral infections such as warts, and possibly the course of certain malignancies such as melanoma. There is a group of disorders such as psoriasis, atopic dermatitis, chronic idiopathic urticaria, alopecia areata and acne that have a stronger psychiatric and psychosocial component as they are often exacerbated by psychosocial stress and are frequently comorbid with major psychiatric syndromes such as depressive illness. Some of the major psychiatric disorders (American Psychiatric Association, 1994) that are encountered in dermatology include mood disorders such as major depressive disorder; anxiety disorders such as obsessive–compulsive disorder (OCD), social phobia, anxiety disorder due to a general medical condition and post-traumatic stress disorder (PTSD); somatoform disorders such as body dysmorphic disorder (BDD); psychotic disorders such as delusional disorder, somatic type encountered in delusions of parasitosis, shared psychotic disorder or folie a deux; and the eating disorders such as anorexia nervosa and bulimia nervosa. The personality disorders, especially the borderline, narcissistic, histrionic and obsessive–compulsive personality types, may be encountered in certain groups of dermatology patients. This chapter reviews some of the more recent literature on the psychiatric comorbidity in dermatological disorders.

The interaction between the skin and the psyche begins in early development and it is important to assess psychiatric pathology in the dermatological patient from a developmental perspective. The common ectodermal origins of the epidermis and the central nervous system suggest that some dermatological and psychiatric disorders share a common origin. The skin is a vital organ of communication and plays a central role in early attachment. The earliest social interactions between the infant and its caregivers occur through the body, especially through touch. Skin disorders during infancy may result in a decrease in the tactile nurturance such as secure holding, massage and hugging that the infant receives from the caregiver. Contact clinging or care by close skin-to-skin touching is a primary factor in maternal–infant bonding and a failure to develop the primary bond has been associated with depression in later life. Inadequate tactile nurturance in early development may also lead to body image problems in later life (Gupta et al., 1995). During adolescence, the impact of a cosmetically disfiguring skin disorder is further confounded by the fact that this life stage is also associated with the high incidence of depression and body image disorders. All these factors can culminate in serious psychiatric reactions including suicide, for instance among some adolescent acne patients. Since the skin remains a powerful medium of communication throughout the life cycle, disfiguring skin conditions at any age can have a significant impact on the quality of life of the patient, which in some cases can result in serious psychiatric morbidity and considerable psychosocial stress.

As the interface between dermatology and psychiatry is often very complex, the dermatological conditions such as psoriasis or acne are often a precipitating or triggering factor in a patient who may be otherwise predisposed genetically to develop a psychiatric disorder such as depressive illness or OCD. Therefore, it may be more appropriate to adopt a multidimensional biopsychosocial (Engel, 1980) approach, which allows for the relative contributions of biological, psychiatric and psychosocial factors when assessing the dermatological patient, as it may not be possible to clearly determine whether a psychiatric syndrome is primary or strictly secondary to the dermatological condition.

Major depressive disorder

Major depressive disorder (American Psychiatric Association, 1994) is one of the most commonly encountered psychiatric disorders in dermatology (Gupta &

Gupta, 1996; Woodruff et al., 1997). Major depressive disorder (Diagnostic and Statistical Manual of Mental Disorders – Fourth Edition (DSM-IV)) (American Psychiatric Association, 1994) is characterised by one or more major depressive episodes. Depression is a recurrent disorder and 50–60% of patients who have experienced one major depressive episode are expected to have a second episode. In about two-thirds of cases the major depressive episode remits completely, and in one-third of the syndrome remits only partially or not at all. Chronic medical conditions (such as chronic recurrent skin disorders) are a known risk factor for more persistent episodes of depression.

A major depressive episode (American Psychiatric Association, 1994) is associated with at least 2 weeks of depressed mood, or loss of interest or pleasure in activities that the patient previously found pleasurable or interesting. In children the depression often manifests as dysphoria and irritability rather than frank depression, and in some adults the most prominent affect may be one of anxiety and agitation rather than sadness and depression. It is important not to misdiagnose these symptoms as being representative of a primary anxiety disorder. The mood changes in depression are accompanied by four or more symptoms that represent a change from the previous functioning of the patient including psychomotor agitation or retardation; difficulties with initiating and maintaining sleep or hypersomnia nearly every day; decrease or increase in appetite; fatigue or loss of energy; feelings of worthlessness, or excessive or inappropriate guilt; indecisiveness or decreased concentrating ability; and recurrent thoughts of death with or without suicidal ideation. Some of these symptoms such as sleep difficulties can complicate other dermatological symptoms like pruritus and difficulties with concentration may interfere with adherence to prescribed treatments. The psychomotor agitation experienced by some patients can be associated with hair pulling, rubbing, scratching or picking of the skin.

Depressive disease is a clinically important feature of psoriasis (Russo et al., 2004). Onset of psoriasis prior to age 40 years has been associated with greater difficulties with the expression of anger (Gupta et al., 1996), a personality trait which may predispose the patient to develop depression and be more vulnerable to psychosocial stressors. Psoriasis-related stress has been associated with greater psychiatric morbidity (Fortune et al., 1997) as patients who feel stigmatised in social situations have higher depression scores. Adult psoriasis patients who experienced greater deprivation of social touch as a result of their psoriasis had higher depression scores than patients who did not feel stigmatised (Gupta et al., 1998). Pruritus, which is reported to be one of the most bothersome features of psoriasis, has been associated with suicide. In psoriasis, severity of pruritus correlates directly with the severity of depressive symptoms (Gupta et al., 1988; Gupta et al., 1994). Improvement in pruritus has been associated with an improvement in depression scores among psoriasis patients (Gupta et al., 1988) and the severity of the skin disorder correlates directly with the severity of depression and frequency of suicidal ideation (Gupta et al., 1993). In a cross-sectional survey, a 2.5% prevalence of suicidal ideation was observed among less severely affected psoriasis outpatients in contrast to a 7.2% suicidal ideation among the more severely affected inpatients with psoriasis (Gupta & Gupta, 1998).

The psychiatric morbidity in acne (Gupta & Gupta, 2001b) is often the most important index of disease severity and often the most important factor in deciding whether or not to institute treatments for the acne, especially in the case of mild-to-moderate disease. The psychiatric morbidity in acne can be severe and comparable to the disability resulting from other chronic disorders such as diabetes and asthma (Mallon et al., 1999). In contrast to psoriasis, the severity of acne does not necessarily correlate with the severity of depression (Aktan et al., 2000; Yazici et al., 2004), as even mild-to-moderate acne has been associated with depression, suicidal ideation (Gupta & Gupta, 1998) and completed suicide (Cotterill & Cunliffe, 1997). Adolescent acne patients who experience problems at school or work and blame it mainly on their acne may be clinically depressed (Gupta et al., 1998). Treatment of both mild-to-moderate non-cystic acne (Gupta et al., 1990) and the treatment of cystic acne with isotretinoin have been associated with an improvement in psychiatric morbidity, including depression (Rubinow et al., 1987). In a cross-sectional survey, a 5.6% prevalence of suicidal ideation was observed among patients with mild-to-moderate non-cystic facial acne (Gupta & Gupta, 1998). The peak incidence of acne is during mid-adolescence, a life stage that is also associated with a high incidence of depressive disease, and body image disorders. This may be one reason why the prevalence of psychiatric morbidity, including depressive disease in even mild-to-moderate acne, is relatively high in some instances.

The association between acne and depression is further confounded by reports of a possible link between isotretinoin, depression, suicidal ideation, suicide attempts and suicide (Lamberg, 1998; Gupta & Gupta, 2001b; Hull & D'Arcy, 2003). A large-scale epidemiological study (Jick et al., 2000) that examined medical databases failed to demonstrate an increased prevalence of depression, suicide or other psychiatric disorders among acne patients who were using isotretinoin versus those who were using other antibiotics. However, in individual case studies, the relation between depression and isotretinoin was confirmed by re-challenging the patient with isotretinoin (Scheinman et al., 1990). A past history of depressive disease does not appear to increase the risk of developing depression when the patient is challenged with isotretinoin, and patients who develop depression with isotretinoin may have previously used the drug with no adverse psychiatric effects (Scheinman et al., 1990). The literature suggests that the association between depression and isotretinoin is a sporadic and idiosyncratic phenomenon.

Depression is encountered in a wide range of other dermatological disorders (Panconesi, 1984; Gupta & Gupta, 1996; Woodruff et al., 1997; Picardi et al., 2000; Gupta & Gupta, 2003; Picardi et al., 2004; Sampogna et al., 2004). Depression may modulate pruritus perception in other pruritic skin disorders such as atopic dermatitis and chronic idiopathic urticaria in addition to psoriasis (Gupta et al., 1994). Higher anxiety and depressive symptoms (Ullman et al., 1977; Hashiro & Okumura, 1998; Kiebert et al., 2002; Zachariae et al., 2004) have been reported in patients with atopic dermatitis. The anxiety may be the feature of an underlying depressive illness in some of these patients. Chronic intractable eczema during childhood may be a sign of a disturbed parent/child relationship (Koblenzer & Koblenzer, 1988); however, a major depressive disorder should be ruled out before a disturbance in the family dynamics is implicated (Allen, 1989). Chronic idiopathic urticaria has been associated with a wide range of psychopathology (Rees, 1957; Czubalski & Rudzki, 1977; Juhlin, 1981; Sheehan-Dare, 1990; Badoux & Levy, 1994) and frequently associated with difficulties with the expression of anger and increased hostility, personality traits which may both predispose the patient to develop depression. Alopecia areata has been associated with depressive disease; however, this association is not a consistent finding across studies. In a survey of 294 alopecia areata patients, the prevalence of major depression was 8.8% (Koo et al., 1994). Another survey of 31 patients with alopecia areata reported a 74% lifetime prevalence of one or more psychiatric disorders with 39% prevalence of major depression (Colon et al., 1991). A study of 32 patients with alopecia areata reported a 66% prevalence of psychiatric comorbidity including generalised anxiety disorder, adjustment disorder and major depressive episodes (Ruiz-Doblado et al., 2003). However, a study of 52 patients with alopecia areata found no significant difference in psychological morbidity between patients and non-clinical controls with no alopecia (Gulec et al., 2004). In this study, the patients with stress-reactive alopecia areata had experienced more major life events (Gulec et al., 2004), supporting the possible role of stress. In another study, patients whose alopecia areata was more reactive to stress also had higher depression scores, suggesting that comorbid depression may render the condition more stress reactive (Gupta et al., 1997).

Some depressed patients may complain of cutaneous dysaesthesias such as pain and burning sensations, for which no physical basis can be identified. These symptoms may represent 'masked depression' or 'depressive equivalents' as some patients lack psychological insight and may deny an underlying depressive disorder (Gupta & Gupta, 1996). Some other patients with primary depressive disease may become preoccupied with relatively minor dermatological problems such as minimal hair loss. More severe depressive disease (American Psychiatric Association, 1994) can present with mood-congruent delusions; for example, of having an incurable skin disease or delusions that their skin is rotting or emitting a foul odour.

The vegetative disturbances associated with depressive disease are a central feature of the syndrome (American Psychiatric Association, 1994). It is well recognised that depressive disorder is accompanied by measurable alterations of circadian rhythms for example, cortisol secretion and the sleep-wake cycle. A commonly encountered clinical feature of circadian rhythm disturbance is the worsening of mood, energy and psychomotor activity early in the day with an improvement during the latter part of the day. Another disturbance of biological rhythm encountered in mood disorders is seasonal worsening of depressive symptoms in some patients, especially during the fall and winter months. The depression-related somatic concerns related to the integumentary system, or symptoms which are related to depression such as pruritus can therefore also manifest a diurnal or seasonal pattern.

Suicide, defined as intentional self-inflicted death, is a central feature of depressive disease and 50% of all persons who commit suicide are depressed (Sadock & Sadock, 2001); 15% of depressed individuals eventually kill themselves and the suicide rate in the USA is 12 per 100,000 (Sadock & Sadock, 2001). Among men the suicide rate peaks after age 45 years and among women after age 65 years (Sadock & Sadock, 2001). After age 75 years, the suicide rate rises in both sexes. Women attempt suicide four times more frequently than men; however, men commit suicide three times more often than women. Currently, there is a rapid rise in suicide rates among males between 15 and 24 years (Sadock & Sadock, 2001). Suicidal behaviour in the adolescent acne patient therefore may not be solely due to the psychosocial impact of the acne.

Obsessive–compulsive disorder

OCD (American Psychiatric Association, 1994) is characterised by recurrent obsessions or compulsions severe enough to be time consuming or cause marked distress or significant impairment. OCD is an anxiety disorder, and some of the compulsive behaviours of OCD may in fact further exacerbate skin disorders that are associated with or exacerbated by anxiety such as atopic dermatitis. Some of the compulsions involve repetitive behaviours such as hand washing, hair plucking, trichotillomania, onychophagia, picking of a minor irregularity in the skin or lesions on the skin and repetitive bathing or scratching (Hatch et al., 1992; Stein & Hollander, 1992; Monti et al., 1998; Calikusu et al., 2003). The patient with OCD feels driven to perform in response to an obsession which, if resisted, produces anxiety. The compulsive scratching of OCD may exacerbate a primary skin disorder such as psoriasis, eczema and other pruritic conditions, or cause flare-ups of acne as in *acne excoriee*. OCD symptoms often result in dermatitis as a result of excessive hand washing and bathing. An overconcern with dermatological symptoms that are not consistent with objective dermatological evaluation may represent underlying OCD in the patient who has difficulty tolerating even a minor imperfection in their complexion and is driven to seek various therapies.

Social phobia (social anxiety disorder)

Social phobia (American Psychiatric Association, 1994) is characterised by a marked or persistent fear of one or more social or performance situations in which the person is exposed to unfamiliar people or to the possible scrutiny of others (American Psychiatric Association, 1994). The individual fears that he or she will act in a way or show anxiety symptoms that will be humiliating or embarrassing. For example, some patients with hyperhydrosis and rosacea often perspire or blush more prominently in embarrassing situations and may develop a social phobia as a result. Exposure to the feared social situation almost always provokes anxiety, which may take the form of a situationally bound panic attack, which in turn also results in an exaggerated autonomic reactivity of the skin. In social phobia the individual recognises that the fear is excessive or unreasonable; however, intense anxiety results if the feared situation is not avoided. The anxious anticipation or distress of the feared social or performance situation interferes significantly with the individual's overall functioning. Social phobia is also encountered in patients with cosmetically disfiguring skin disorders (Kent & Keohane, 2001) such as psoriasis and acne (Gupta & Gupta, 1996; Woodruff et al., 1997), especially those who have been teased or ridiculed about their skin disorder at some time earlier in their lives. Some patients with chronic acne whose acne had interfered with their socialisation during their adolescence continue to experience social anxiety in later life when they no longer have the acne, because of the long-term impact of having to live with acne during developmentally critical periods of life such as adolescence (Kellett & Gawkrodger, 1999). Patients with social phobia are typically under-diagnosed because the very nature of their disorder prevents them from attending clinics and doctors offices where they have to face large numbers of relatively unfamiliar people.

Post-traumatic stress disorder

PTSD-related symptoms tend to be under-recognised in dermatology (Woodruff et al., 1997). The central clinical features of PTSD (American Psychiatric Association, 1994) include the persistent re-experience of extremely traumatic or stressful life experiences or life events, which can manifest as recurrent and intrusive thoughts, dreams, flashbacks or physical symptoms. There is a persistent avoidance of stimuli associated with the trauma and this can manifest as dissociative symptoms.

PTSD secondary to childhood neglect and abuse, especially sexual abuse, is often the underlying psychiatric pathology in dermatological patients who self-induce their lesions. PTSD is often complicated by substance abuse disorders and this often becomes the main focus in treatment. When dissociative symptoms are a prominent feature of the PTSD, the patient may not have recollection of the fact that they self-induced their lesions (Shelley, 1981; Gupta et al., 2000) and may be misdiagnosed as malingerers or attentions seekers and the central role of psychological trauma is often overlooked. PTSD, dissociation and self-injury (Gupta et al., 2000) can be the underlying psychiatric disturbance in some cases of trichotillomania and dermatitis artefacta or may complicate the course of other dermatological conditions such as *acne excoriee* or the exacerbation of psoriatic lesions secondary to the Koebner phenomenon.

Tactile nurturance, consisting of secure holding and hugging, is essential for the formation of a healthy body image (Gupta et al., 1995), including cutaneous body image. When there is neglect and/or abuse in early life, the infant does not experience healthy tactile nurturance and may be predisposed to developing body image problems in later life. It has been observed that a perceived lack of adequate tactile nurturance is associated with body image problems (Gupta et al., 1995). A patient with a significant history of trauma or neglect may therefore present with dissatisfaction with their body image including cutaneous body image.

BDD and other body image pathologies

BDD presents as a preoccupation with an imagined defect in appearance; or if a slight anomaly is present, the individual's concern is excessive (American Psychiatric Association, 1994). BDD is also referred to as dysmorphophobia and 'dermatological non-disease' (Cotterill, 1981) in the dermatological literature. In one study 8.8% of patients with mild acne had BDD (Uzun et al., 2003). The complaints in BDD commonly involve imagined or slight flaws of the face or head such as thinning hair, acne, wrinkles, scars, vascular markings, paleness or redness of the complexion, swelling, facial disproportion or asymmetry, or excessive facial hair. The most common areas of concern involve the skin and hair. Some associated features of BDD include repetitive behaviours such as excessive grooming behaviour. This may manifest as excessive hair combing, hair removal, hair picking or picking of the skin, or ritualised make-up application. The main purpose of the repetitive behaviour is to improve or hide the perceived defect in the appearance. Many individuals may camouflage their perceived defect or deformity with make-up or clothing or hair. Most individuals with BDD experience marked distress over their supposed deformity and feelings of self-consciousness over their 'defect', which often leads to vocational and social impairment. In some instances BDD can be life threatening as patients may resort to extreme behaviours to deal with a perceived defect in their appearance, for example they may use razor blades or knives to remove these 'defects'. In some patients the preoccupation with a minimal or imagined 'defect' in appearance can reach delusional proportions.

Patients with eating disorders such as anorexia nervosa and bulimia nervosa often present with excessive concerns about their cutaneous body image in addition to concerns about their weight and shape (Gupta & Gupta, 2001a). The eating disorders can be associated with a wide range of dermatological (Gupta et al., 1987; Gupta & Gupta, 2000) complications related to starvation, bingeing and purging, abuse of laxatives and other related symptoms (American Psychiatric Association, 1994). Acne has a peak incidence during mid-adolescence, a life stage that is associated with a high incidence of eating disorders. In some vulnerable adolescents even mild acne may exacerbate or precipitate an eating disorder such as bulimia nervosa (Gupta et al., 1987; Gupta & Gupta, 2000). The endocrine changes associated with binge eating may cause a flare-up of acne (Gupta et al., 1992), which is frequently observed in patients with eating disorders (Gupta & Gupta, 2000). In these patients the disfigurement caused by the self-excoriation of acne lesions can serve as a 'protective device' or excuse for avoiding some of the social and vocational tasks of adolescence and young adulthood (Cotterill, 1981). Patients with *acne excoriee des jeunes filles* present with psychological dynamics that are very similar to the dynamics encountered in eating disorders such as difficulties in coping with the developmental tasks of young adulthood. The body image pathologies in conjunction with immature coping mechanisms often result in relatively intractable symptoms in the patients who use their skin lesions as a 'protective device' and a coping mechanism.

Delusional disorder and other psychotic symptoms

The essential feature of delusional disorder (American Psychiatric Association, 1994) is the presence of one or more non-bizarre delusions that persist for at least 1 month. A delusion is defined as a false belief, based on faulty or incorrect interpretation of external reality that is not consistent with the patients' cultural background or intelligence and cannot be corrected by reasoning. A delusion that is frequently referenced in the dermatological literature is delusion of parasitosis (Driscoll et al., 1993). The delusion may be associated with tactile or olfactory hallucinations that are related to the theme of the delusion; for instance, a crawling sensation under the skin in association with delusions of parasitosis, or a delusion that one is emitting a foul odour from an orifice of the body. This can occur in conjunction with delusions of reference where the patient believes that everyone around him is talking about the odour that he is emitting. Certain hallucinations related to touch may in part be related to an organic brain syndrome or peripheral degenerative changes that may cause some cutaneous dysaesthesias. A delusional disorder may coexist with a major depressive episode where the patient experiences delusions that are congruent with his or her depressed mood, and typically represent a more severe form of depressive disease. BDD is often associated with delusions of disfigurement. If the delusion or hallucination becomes more bizarre and if they are clearly implausible and not derived from normal life experience (e.g. a complaint that aliens are putting electricity through the body and causing the patient to feel a stinging sensation in the skin) the diagnosis of schizophrenia should be considered.

Personality disorders

The personality disorders (American Psychiatric Association, 1994) are defined as an enduring pattern of inner experience and behaviour that is pervasive across a wide range of personal and social situations and deviate markedly from the expectations of the individual's culture. The personality disorders that are most frequently encountered in dermatology include Borderline, Narcissistic and Histrionic personality disorders which all fall in the 'Cluster B' (American Psychiatric Association, 1994) category in the DSM-IV and Obsessive–compulsive personality disorder (which is categorised in 'Cluster C'). Borderline personality disorder is associated with a pattern of instability in interpersonal relationships, affects and self-image, and impulsive behaviours. Such patients are often 'difficult' as their instability in interpersonal relationships and self-image are also manifested in their relationship with their dermatologists and other health care providers. Such patients often try to 'split' or play one professional against the other, and at times may be very unreasonable, manipulative and demanding. The borderline patient is also prone to impulsive self-harm such as cutting of the skin. Narcissistic personality disorder presents with a pattern of grandiosity, need for admiration and often a lack of empathy for others. Some such patients may place an inordinate importance on their appearance and the approval of others, and face a psychiatric crisis including suicidal ideation, when faced with a cosmetically disfiguring skin disorder or the normal changes of aging. The patient with a Histrionic personality disorder presents with excessive emotionality and are attention seeking. Some such patients, who have very immature coping mechanisms, may self-induce skin lesions to get attention. This can be the case in dermatitis artefacta or some patients with *acne excoriee des jeunes filles*. In Obsessive–compulsive personality disorder there is a pattern of preoccupation with orderliness, perfectionism and control. This may be a feature in patients with compulsive behaviours such as compulsive washing and picking of the skin, or patients with excessive body image concerns where the patient is bothered by a minor or nonexistent 'imperfection' in their skin.

Conclusion

The interface between psychiatry and dermatology is multidimensional and begins in early development. The skin is a vital organ of communication and the earliest social interactions between the infant and its caregivers occur via the body, especially through touch. A disruption in tactile nurturance, for example, as a result of a skin disorder during infancy or due to childhood abuse and/or neglect can be associated with serious psychiatric morbidity in later life including major depressive disorder, body image pathologies, a tendency to self-injure and dissociative states when there is significant psychological trauma present in association with the neglect. The importance of the skin in social communication is further exemplified during adolescence when the development of a cosmetically disfiguring skin disorder such as acne can be associated with depression, suicidal ideation and body image disorders including eating disorders. The role of the skin as an organ of communication remains important throughout the life cycle, as the development of a disfiguring skin condition at any life stage can have a significant impact on the quality of life of the patient. In certain conditions such as acne and psoriasis, the psychiatric comorbidity and the impact of the skin disorder on the quality of life of the patient are often the most important component of the overall morbidity associated with the skin condition.

Psychiatric disorders in the dermatological patient are generally assumed to be secondary to the skin disorder; however, in some instances they may be primary and/or have a direct impact on the course of the dermatological symptoms. Pruritus severity in psoriasis and atopic dermatitis has been noted to correlate directly with the severity of depressive symptoms in the patient, suggesting that depression may modulate pruritus perception. Depressive disease is one of the most frequently encountered psychiatric disorders in dermatology and may be a feature of a wide range of conditions including psoriasis, acne, chronic idiopathic urticaria and atopic dermatitis. Depressive symptoms may also present as somatic equivalents, for instance cutaneous dysaesthesias for which no physical basis can be identified. Psoriasis and acne have been associated with suicidal ideation and suicide. In psoriasis the frequency of suicidal ideation generally increases with increasing psoriasis severity; however among acne patients, the severity of the skin lesions and frequency of suicidal ideation do not show a consistent relationship, as even mild-to-moderate acne has been associated with depression, suicidal ideation and completed suicide.

Some of the other psychiatric syndromes in dermatology include OCD which may manifest as repetitive hand washing or bathing, trichotillomania, onychophagia, neurotic excoriations or an excessive concern about a minor or imagined 'defect' in the skin. Social phobia or social anxiety disorder can be a feature of a wide range of cosmetically disfiguring conditions or conditions that become more visible when the patient is autonomically aroused such as rosacea and hyperhydrosis. PTSD is often under-recognised and may be an underlying problem in the self-induced dermatoses such as trichotillomania and dermatitis artefacta. BDD or dysmorphophobia is often encountered in patients who present with an excessive concern about a minimal or imagined dermatological problem such as minimal acne, wrinkles or vascular markings.

Overall, it is important to evaluate and manage the psychiatric comorbidity in the dermatological patient, as they can contribute towards a large proportion of the overall morbidity associated with the skin disorder and usually have a significant impact on the quality of life of the patient. In some instances, the psychiatric comorbidity such as depressive disease can have an adverse impact on dermatological aspects of the disorder due to poor adherence to treatment or a possible direct effect on certain symptoms such as pruritus. Certain body image pathologies may predispose the patient to overestimate the severity of their dermatological symptom, which may culminate in excessive concerns about minor problems or patient dissatisfaction with treatment outcome. It is therefore increasingly recognised that an improvement in psychiatric comorbidity is an important measure of treatment outcome for a wide range of dermatological patients.

REFERENCES

Aktan, S., Ozmen, E., & Sanli, B. (2000). Anxiety, depression, and nature of acne vulgaris in adolescents. *International Journal of Dermatology*, **39**, 354–357.

Allen, A.D. (1989). Intractable atopic eczema suggests major affective disorder: poor parenting is secondary (letter). *Archives of Dermatology*, **125**, 567–568.

American Psychiatric Association Committee on Nomenclature and Statistics (1994). *Diagnostic and Statistical Manual of Mental Disorders*, 4th edn. Washington, DC: American Psychiatric Association.

Badoux, A., & Levy, D.A. (1994). Psychologic symptoms in asthma and chronic urticaria. *Annals of Allergy*, **72**, 229–234.

Calikusu, C., Yucel, B., Polat, A., & Baykal, C. (2003). The relation of psychogenic excoriation with psychiatric disorders: a comparative study. *Comprehensive Psychiatry*, **44**, 256–261.

Colon, E.A., Popkin, M.K., Callies, A.L., Dessert, N.J., & Hordinsky, M.K. (1991). Lifetime prevalence of psychiatric disorders in patients with alopecia areata. *Comprehensive Psychiatry*, **32**, 245–251.

Cotterill, J.A. (1981). Dermatologic non-disease: a common and potentially fatal disturbance of cutaneous body image. *British Journal of Dermatology*, **104**, 611.

Cotterill, J.A., & Cunliffe, W.J. (1997). Suicide in dermatological patients. *British Journal of Dermatology*, **137**(2), 246–250.

Czubalski, K., & Rudzki, E. (1977). Neuropsychic factors in physical urticaria. *Dermatologica*, **154**, 1–4.

Driscoll, M.S., Rothe, M.J., Grant-Kels, J.M., & Hale, M.S. (1993). Delusional parasitosis: a dermatologic, psychiatric and pharmacologic approach. *Journal of American Academy of Dermatology*, **29**, 1023–1033.

Engel, G.L. (1980). The clinical application of the biopsychosocial model. *American Journal of Psychiatry*, **137**, 535–544.

Fortune, D.G., Main, C.J., O'Sullivan, T.M., & Griffiths, C.E. (1997). Quality of life in patients with psoriasis: the contribution of clinical variables and psoriasis-specific stress. *British Journal of Dermatology*, **137**, 755–760.

Gulec, A.T., Tanriverdi, N., Duru, C., Saray, Y., & Akcali, C. (2004). The role of psychological factors in alopecia areata and the impact of the disease on the quality of life. *International Journal of Dermatology*, **43**, 352–356.

Gupta, M.A., & Gupta, A.K. (1996). Psychodermatology: an update. *Journal of American Academy of Dermatology*, **34**, 1030–1046.

Gupta, M.A., & Gupta, A.K. (1998). Depression and suicidal ideation in dermatology patients with acne, alopecia areata, atopic dermatitis and psoriasis. *British Journal of Dermatology*, **139(5)**, 846–850.

Gupta, M.A., & Gupta, A.K. (2000). Dermatological complications. *European Eating Disorders Review*, **8(2)**, 134–143.

Gupta, M.A., & Gupta, A.K. (2001a). Dissatisfaction with skin appearance among patients with eating disorders and non-clinical controls. *British Journal of Dermatology*, **145**, 110–113.

Gupta, M.A., & Gupta, A.K. (2001b). The psychological comorbidity in acne. *Clinical Dermatology*, **19**, 360–363.

Gupta, M.A., & Gupta, A.K. (2003). Psychiatric and psychological comorbidity in patients with dermatologic disorders. *American Journal of Clinical Dermatology*, **4(12)**, 833–842.

Gupta, M.A., Gupta, A.K., & Haberman, H.F. (1987). Dermatologic signs in anorexia nervosa and bulimia nervosa. *Archives of Dermatology*, **123**, 1386–1390.

Gupta, M.A., Gupta, A.K., Kirkby, S., Weiner, H.K., Mace, T.M., Schork, N.J., Johnson, E.H., Ellis, C.N., & Voorhees, J.J. (1988). Pruritus in psoriasis: a prospective study of some psychiatric and dermatologic correlates. *Archives of Dermatology*, **124**, 1052–1057.

Gupta, M.A., Gupta, A.K., Schork, N.J., Ellis, C.N., & Voorhees, J.J. (1990). Psychiatric aspects of the treatment of mild to moderate facial acne: some preliminary observations. *International Journal of Dermatology*, **29(10)**, 719–721.

Gupta, M.A., Gupta, A.K., Ellis, C.N., & Voorhees, J.J. (1992). Bulimia nervosa and acne may be related: a case report. *Canadian Journal of Psychiatry*, **37**, 58–61.

Gupta, M.A., Schork, N.J., Gupta, A.K., Kirkby, S., & Ellis, C.N. (1993). Suicidal ideation in psoriasis. *International Journal of Dermatology*, **32**, 188–190.

Gupta, M.A., Gupta, A.K., Schork, N.J., & Ellis, C.N. (1994). Depression modulates pruritus perception: a study of pruritus in psoriasis, atopic dermatitis, and chronic idiopathic urticaria. *Psychosomatic Medicine*, **56**, 36–40.

Gupta, M.A., Gupta, A.K., Schork, N.J., & Watteel, G.N. (1995). Perceived touch deprivation and body image: some observations among eating disordered and non-clinical subjects. *Journal of Psychosomatic Research*, **39**, 459–464.

Gupta, M.A., Gupta, A.K., & Watteel, G. (1996). Early onset (<age 40 years) psoriasis is associated with greater psychopathology than late onset psoriasis. *Acta Dermato-Venereologica*, **76**, 464–466.

Gupta, M.A., Gupta, A.K., & Watteel, G.N. (1997). Stress and alopecia areata: a psychodermatologic study. *Acta Dermato-Venereologica (Stockholm)*, **77**, 296–298.

Gupta, M.A., Gupta, A.K., & Watteel, G.N. (1998). Perceived deprivation of social touch in psoriasis is associated with greater psychological morbidity: an index of the stigma experience in dermatologic disorders. *Cutis*, **61**, 339–342.

Gupta, M.A., Johnson, A.M., & Gupta, A.K. (1998). The development of an acne quality of life scale: reliability, validity, and relation to subjective acne severity in mild to moderated acne vulgaris. *Acta Dermato-Venereologica*, **78(6)**, 451–456.

Gupta, M.A., Gupta, A.K., Chandarana, P.C., & Johnson, A.M. (2000). Dissociative symptoms and self-induced dermatoses: a preliminary empirical study (Abstract). *Psychosomatic Medicine*, **62**, 116.

Hashiro, M., & Okumura, M. (1998). The relationship between the psychological and immunological in patients with atopic dermatitis. *Journal of Dermatological Science*, **16(3)**, 231–235.

Hatch, M.L., Paradis, C., Friedman, S., Popkin, M., & Shalita, A.R. (1992). Obsessive–compulsive disorder in patients with chronic pruritic conditions: case studies and discussion. *Journal of American Academy of Dermatology*, **26**, 549–551.

Hull, P.R., & D'Arcy, C. (2003). Isotretinoin use and subsequent depression and suicide: presenting the evidence. *American Journal of Clinical Dermatology*, **4**, 493–505.

Jick, S.S., Kremers, H.M., & Vasilakis-Scaramozza, C. (2000). Isotretinoin use and risk of depression, psychotic symptoms, suicide and attempted suicide. *Archives of Dermatology*, **136**, 1231–1236.

Juhlin, L. (1981). Recurrent urticaria: clinical investigation of 330 patients. *British Journal of Dermatology*, **104**, 369–381.

Kellett, S.C., & Gawkrodger, D.J. (1999). The psychological and emotional impact of acne and the effect of treatment with isotretinoin. *British Journal of Dermatology*, **140(2)**, 273–282.

Kent, G., & Keohane, S. (2001). Social anxiety and disfigurement: the moderating effects of fear of negative evaluation and past experiences. *British Journal of Clinical Psychology*, **40**, 23–34.

Kiebert, G., Sorensen, S.V., Revicki, D., Fagan, S.C., Doyle, J.J., Cohen, J., & Fivenson, D. (2002). Atopic dermatitis is associated with a decrement in health-related quality of life. *International Journal of Dermatology*, **41**, 151–158.

Koblenzer, C.S., & Koblenzer, P.J. (1988). Chronic intractable atopic eczema. *Archives of Dermatology*, **124**, 1673–1677.

Koo, J.Y.M., Shellow, W.V., Hallman, C.P., & Edwards, J.E. (1994). Alopecia areata and increased prevalence of psychiatric disorders. *International Journal of Dermatology*, **33**, 849–850.

Lamberg, L. (1998). Acne drug depression warnings highlight need for expert care. *Journal of American Medical Association*, **279**, 1057.

Mallon, E., Newton, J.N., Klassen, A., Stewart-Brown, S.L., Ryan, T.J., & Finlay, A.Y. (1999). The quality of life in acne: a comparison with general medical conditions using generic questionnaires. *British Journal of Dermatology*, **140(4)**, 672–676.

Monti, M., Sambvani, N., & Sacrini, F. (1998). Obsessive–compulsive disorders in dermatology. *Journal of European Academy of Dermatology and Venereology*, **11**, 103–108.

Panconesi, P. (1984). Psychosomatic dermatology. *Clinical Dermatology*, **2**, 94–179.

Picardi, A., Abeni, D., & Melchi, C.F. et al. (2000). Psychiatric morbidity in dermatological out-patients: an issue to be recognized. *British Journal of Dermatology*, **143**, 983–991.

Picardi, A., Abeni, D., Renzi, C., Braga, M., Melchi, C.F., & Pasquini, P. (2003). Treatment out-come and incidence of psychiatric disorders in dermatologic out-patients. *Journal of European Academy of Dermatology and Venereology*, **17**, 155–159.

Picardi, A., Amerio, P., Baliva, G., Barbieri, C., Teofoli, P., Bolli, S., Salvatori, V., Mazzotti, E., Pasquini, P., & Abeni, D. (2004). Recognition of depressive and anxiety disorders in dermato-logical outpatients. *Acta Dermato-Venereologica*, **84**, 213–217.

Rees, L. (1957). An aetiological study of chronic urticaria and angioneurotic oedema. *Journal of Psychosomatic Research*, **2**, 172–189.

Rubinow, D.R., Peck, G.L., Squillace, K.M., & Gantt, G.G. (1987). Reduced anxiety and depres-sion in cystic acne patients after successful treatment with oral isotretinoin. *Journal of American Academy of Dermatology*, **17(1)**, 25–32.

Ruiz-Doblado, S., Carrizosa, A., & Garcia-Hernandez, M.J. (2003). Alopecia areata: psychiatric comorbidity and adjustment to illness. *International Journal of Dermatology*, **42**, 434–437.

Russo, P.A., Ilchef, R., & Cooper, A.J. (2004). Psychiatric morbidity in psoriasis: a review. *Australasian Journal of Dermatology*, **45**, 155–159.

Sadock, B.J., & Sadock, V.A. (2001). *Kaplan and Sadock's Pocket Book of Clinical Psychiatry*, 3rd edn. Philadelphia: Lippincott Williams and Wilkins, pp. 261–274.

Sampogna, F., Picardi, A., Chren, M.M., Melchi, C.F., Pasquini, P., Masini, C., & Abeni, D. (2004). Association between poorer quality of life and psychiatric morbidity in patients with different dermatological conditions. *Psychosomatic Medicine*, **66**, 620–640.

Scheinman, P.L., Peck, G.L., Rubinow, D.R., DiGiovanni, J.J., Abangan, D.L., & Ravin, P.D. (1990). Acute depression from isotretinoin. *Journal of American Academy of Dermatology*, **22**, 1112–1114.

Sheehan-Dare, R.A., Henderson, M.J., & Cotterill, J.A. (1990). Anxiety and depression in patients with chronic urticaria and generalized pruritus. *British Journal of Dermatology*, **123**, 769–774.

Shelley, W.B. (1981). Dermatitis artefacta induced in a patient by one of her multiple personal-ities. *British Journal of Dermatology*, **105**, 587–589.

Stein, D.J., & Hollander, E. (1992). Dermatology and conditions related to obsessive–compulsive disorder. *Journal of American Academy of Dermatology*, **26**, 237–242.

Ullman, K.C., Moore, R.W., & Reidy, M. (1977). Atopic eczema: a clinical psychiatric study. *Journal of Asthma Research*, **14**, 91–99.

Uzun, O., Basoglu, C., Akar, A., Cansever, A., Ozsahin, A., Cetin, M., & Ebrinc S. (2003). Body dysmorphic disorder in patients with acne. *Comprehensive Psychiatry*, **44**, 415–419.

Woodruff, P.W.R., Higgins, E.M., Du Vivier, A.W.P., & Wessely, S. (1997). Psychiatric illness in patients referred to a dermatology–psychiatry clinic. *General Hospital Psychiatry*, **19**, 29–35.

Yazici, K., Baz, K., Yazici, A.E., Kokturk, A., Tot, S., Demirseren, D., & Buturak, V. (2004). Disease-specific quality of life is associated with anxiety and depression in patients with acne. *Journal of European Academy of Dermatology and Venereology*, **18**, 435–439.

Zachariae, R., Zachariae, C., Ibsen, H.H., Mortensen, J.T., & Wulf, H.C. (2004). Psychological symptoms and quality of life of dermatology outpatients and hospitalized dermatology patients. *Acta Dermato-Venereologica*, **84**, 205–212.

4

Stigmatisation and skin conditions

Gerry Kent

It can be argued that all research on stigma and stigmatisation is a footnote to the sociologist Erving Goffman. In a few short, elegantly written books (e.g. Goffman, 1968), he provided a wealth of ideas and insights, giving much inspiration to work on this topic. Goffman defined a 'stigma' as a mark or sign that not only sets a person apart from others but also leads to their devaluation. He distinguished between three types of stigma: 'tribal identity' (such as race, gender or religion); 'character blemishes' (such as mental illness or addiction); and what he called 'abominations of the body'. Although today we would not wish to use such terms as 'defects', 'abnormalities' or 'flaws' to describe the bodies of people with physical differences, Goffman quite sensitively discussed the issues faced by people whose appearance or function has been compromised in some way.

One of Goffman's central ideas was that the mark or sign comes to take on 'master' status, becoming the most important characteristic of the affected individual. This is illustrated by the following description, given by a person with psoriasis. He is recalling a time when his psoriasis took on more importance in the eyes of others than his more relevant sporting skills and efforts:

'As a schoolboy sportsman I was once called names when going for a shower after an important game. I had made an important contribution in winning but was made to feel an outcast because I was suffering with psoriasis on my shins at the time'.

Since Goffman's seminal work, there have been several collections of essays (e.g. Jones et al., 1984; Heatherton et al., 2000) that cover research on stigma from a general psychological perspective. The aim of this chapter is to review the research on stigma and stigmatisation as it relates to dermatological conditions. The work has been conducted with people with a variety of skin conditions, including vitiligo, psoriasis, port wine stains and eczema. The chapter aims to answer six questions:

1 What types of stigmatisation do people encounter?.
2 What is the nature of these experiences?
3 Why does stigmatisation occur?

4 What are the effects of stigmatisation?

5 Why does stigmatisation matter?

6 How might stigmatisation be reduced?

A seventh section considers future research possibilities.

What types of stigmatisation do people encounter?

People with dermatological conditions often claim that their main difficulties arise from others' reactions to their disease, rather than the disease itself (e.g. Rapp, 1999). Perceptions of stigmatisation are common amongst those with a visible skin difference. For example, Gupta et al. (1998) found that 26% of their patients with psoriasis reported that they had experienced an episode when someone made an effort not to touch them because of their psoriasis. Ginsburg and Link (1989) also explored feelings of stigmatisation in people with psoriasis. They asked patients to complete a questionnaire containing 33 items covering a range of possible feelings and beliefs about how other people react to their psoriasis. A factor analysis indicated that beliefs about stigmatisation could be grouped into six dimensions: anticipation of rejection (e.g. 'I feel physically unattractive and sexually unattractive when the psoriasis is bad'); feelings of being flawed (e.g. 'I often think that others think that psoriasis patients are dirty'); sensitivity to the opinions of others (e.g. 'Sometimes I feel an outcast because of my psoriasis'); secretiveness (e.g. 'I do my best to keep family members I do not live with from knowing that I have psoriasis'); and the more positive dimension, attitudes which correlated negatively with the others (e.g. 'If my child were to have psoriasis I think he or she could develop his or her potential just as though he or she did not have it'). One of the most important predictors of such beliefs was a previous experience of rejection. Similar results were found in a German version of the questionnaire (Schmid-Ott et al., 1996).

Such perceptions and beliefs are not due to over-sensitivity. A number of experimental studies have demonstrated that people with disfiguring skin conditions encounter stigmatisation. For example, Kleck and Strenta (1980) compared reactions to a confederate of the experimenters when the confederate either had an unblemished face or had an artificial scar applied to a cheek. Clearly, other people reacted to the confederate quite differently under the two experimental conditions. They were more likely to judge the confederates behaviour negatively when a scar had been applied to the face. Stigmatisation can be more subtle than this. Rumsey et al. (1982) used make-up so it seemed that a person waiting at a traffic light had either a port wine stain to one side of the face, had an accident to the same side (as indicated by a bandage), or had an unblemished face. Other people waiting at the light stood further away from the confederate when he had a port wine stain, and were less likely to stand on the affected side. People are likely to avoid sitting beside someone whose appearance has been changed due to a port wine stain (Houston & Bull, 1994).

Thus, stigmatisation can occur in a variety of ways. It is possible to distinguish between two types of negative experience: enacted and vicarious stigmatisation. Enacted stigma refers to a direct negative experience, where a person is explicitly rejected on the basis of their mark. For example, Kent and Keohane (2001) asked people with psoriasis to describe an event that made them more concerned about their appearance. Two examples are provided:

'Many years ago, on a very hot day, I removed my cardigan in a café and, after using their toilets I washed my hands and dried them on a roller tower. A young woman said to her friend "Don't use that towel – that woman's just used it". The memory of that day is as vivid now as when it happened. I wanted to curl up and die'.

'When I went to the swimming baths many years ago and two women started pointing at my body and made it obvious that they thought I had something that was catching'.

But other types of stigmatisation might also occur. Vicarious stigmatisation occurs when a person sees someone else experience enacted stigma. Bandura (1977) argued that we gather much information about our environment by watching the experiences of other people. We expect to be treated in a similar fashion to others, depending on the extent to which we are alike or behave in a similar fashion. Examples of this are:

'A new work colleague said that her friend had psoriasis on her elbows and arms, not as bad as mine and she was turned down for a job as a staff nurse in Accident and Emergency somewhere and that she finds it very difficult to get a job'.

'The attitude of a child towards a girl who suffered with psoriasis at school when I was a child at school. She was the butt of all jokes. Regarded as being unclean and if you touched her you caught it'.

Third, although not strictly an instance of stigmatisation because there was no apparent explicit rejection, the following description also provides a powerful example of being marked and devalued by others. In this instance, people working in the shop apparently felt that it was acceptable to treat the person as a curiosity because of their psoriasis:

'When trying on a dress the shop assistant came in, took one look at me and said "Oh, dear" and walked back out again. I then had several shop assistants come in just to look. This of course caused me great embarrassment and I don't like trying on dresses now'.

Finally, though not explored in any detail, it seems that people with skin diseases can stigmatise themselves, being rejecting of their appearance and assuming that others will react in a similar fashion. Wahl et al. (2002) used grounded theory to interview 22 people who had been hospitalised because of their psoriasis. Some of these respondents had a strongly negative view of their skin:

'I think it's disgusting to look at, so other people must feel the same way. I tell myself that others think it is just as disgusting as I do. After all, they have the same eyes and feelings in their hands.' (Wahl et al. (2002), p. 254)

What is the nature of these experiences?

It is surprising that there is so little research on the exact nature of stigmatising experiences. We need a better understanding of what stigmatisation actually looks like, the circumstances under which it occurs and the characteristics of those who do the stigmatising. As noted already, stigmatisation varies along some dimension of explicitness. When Kent and Keohane (2001) performed a content analysis on the situations that led people to be more concerned about their appearance, the experiences could be reliably placed into two categories. Some examples of the first category have been given and there was little ambiguity about the intention or content of the rejection in these examples. Other examples included the following:

'Once when I was catching a bus in the summertime I had on a short skirt and I heard an elderly man and woman say that my legs looked disgusting and I should wear trousers or something so that no one would "catch" it from me'.

'When my daughter was very young she once would not touch me. This was when I had a lot of psoriasis'.

However, and again, the behaviour and the experience can be more subtle. Many people whose appearance is visibly different from others find that staring and intrusive questioning can cause embarrassment and can be an indication that there is 'something wrong' with them:

'If I wear short-sleeve blouses and my arms are uncovered people always ask what is wrong with my skin'.

'Some children commented out loudly on my skin problem while I was on holiday and in the swimming pool and were reprimanded by their parents, which emphasised the incident'.

These are only preliminary attempts to understand the nature of stigmatising experiences. As discussed below, such experiences have significant effects on well-being and so they deserve deeper analysis. It would also be possible to gather data on who expresses these types of behaviour, since the relationship with the stigmatiser may well be important. People with visible differences often say that they tend to encounter stigmatisation from strangers, rather than friends and family, and perhaps friends and family can provide counterbalancing support and acceptance. Age may likewise be important since children often make uncensored remarks.

Why does stigmatisation occur?

This central question has been given a variety of answers. Goffman originally argued that it occurred because of some threat to orderly social interaction. From a sociological point of view, deviations from predictability in social encounters pose a threat to the smooth running of society and there is some evidence that this is part of the answer (Albrecht et al., 1982).

Another possibility involves attribution theory, particularly beliefs about the cause of the condition (Weiner et al., 1988). It seems that people are more likely to be stigmatised if they are seen as having control over the onset or maintenance of their condition (Weiner et al., 1988; Crandall & Moriarty, 1995; Martini & Page, 1998). This idea is particularly relevant to understanding the stigmatisation experienced by people who have nicotine or alcohol dependence, but perhaps also to acne since there is a widespread belief that a poor diet and an unhealthy lifestyle can contribute to its development. The Just World Hypothesis is related to attributions. This is the notion that negative events occur to people because of retributive justice for their actions (Lerner & Miller, 1978). That is, people get what they deserve; if someone has a skin disease they must have done something to merit their appearance.

Another approach to understanding stigmatisation is based on the 'beautiful is good' stereotype. There is considerable evidence for the suggestion that attractive people are viewed differently than unattractive people (Dion et al., 1972; Eagly et al., 1991). Attractive people tend to be seen more positively on a wide variety of dimensions, including intelligence, warmth and social competence, a view that develops in children while they are quite young. The notion that the converse also holds (i.e. that people with disfiguring conditions are perceived as 'bad') has not been tested directly, but media and literary portrayals that often equate evil with such skin conditions as scarring would suggest that a connection of this kind is often made.

It seems likely that all of these ideas have power in explaining stigmatisation across a variety of conditions. A common thread throughout is the possibility that a person with a mark poses some kind of threat to personal or social well-being. There might be a threat to orderly social interaction, perhaps, or that a person is in some way responsible for their condition and should therefore be ostracised as punishment. These beliefs could be operating out of consciousness and awareness.

For dermatological conditions, however, there could be a more direct type of threat – a threat to physical health. There is a growing consensus that stigmatisation has an evolutionary origin because, in our species' past, avoidance of potential threats had advantages for survival. The evolutionary explanation has been outlined by Kurzban and Leary (2001). They argue that this approach to stigmatisation provides a parsimonious and elegant explanation over a wide range of conditions and behaviours, but it might be particularly relevant to skin conditions. As noted above, people with psoriasis and vitiligo can often cite instances when someone avoided making physical contact or touching any object they have used. Such examples lend themselves to understanding stigmatisation and rejection of those with skin conditions in terms of potential contagion. Many people with vitiligo and psoriasis complain that others often do not understand the nature or causes of their conditions, and assume that they might be 'catching'.

Rozin and Fallon (1987) summarise their view that disgust has an evolutionary origin, designed to protect the person from contamination. Their analysis includes a description of the typical expressions of disgust – a characteristic facial express and physical distancing – mirroring the reactions reported above. Rozin and Fallon argue that disgust develops during the first 8 months of life.

What effects does stigmatisation have?

A fourth issue concerns the meaning and effects of stigmatisation on the targeted person. It is clear that such experiences can have a profound effect. In the Kent and Keohane study described above, some of the experiences occurred many years previously, yet were still very fresh in the mind. Indeed, some of the events could be characterised as being almost traumatic:

'As a child I remember parents taking their children away from me at a paddling pool. "Don't play with her" was a memorable comment'.

It seems that stigmatisation can result in significant changes in the ways that targeted people see themselves and, especially, the way they see their social environment. Kent (2002) argued that the effects of these events can be best understood in terms of a cognitive–behavioural model, in which anxiety schema develop after such experiences. The term 'schema' refers to a mental representation of the self and the environment that serves to organise and process incoming information. In this context, incoming information is scanned for indications of threat and the possibility of rejection due to appearance. A kind of 'rejection sensitivity' can develop. The person becomes vigilant for the presence of further stigmatisation, can interpret neutral events as stigmatising, and because of feelings of shame (Gilbert, 2000), attempts to conceal their appearance from others (Smart & Wegner, 1999).

In many respects this notion of anxiety schema is similar to Jacoby's (1994) idea of 'felt stigma' – the expectation that one could be subject to stigmatisation at any time. Kent (1999) adapted the Ginsburg and Link (1989) questionnaire for people with vitiligo. He found a range of statistically significant correlations, with felt stigma being related to scores on: the General Health Questionnaire, a quality of life measure designed for dermatological patients (the DQLI, Finlay & Khan, 1994), self-esteem and a checklist of emotional symptoms. Kent also asked respondents to give a description of any events in which having vitiligo had influenced their lives in some way over the previous 3 weeks. An instance of enacted stigma was described by only 8.6% of the respondents, whereas an instance of felt stigma was described by 38.6% of respondents (the remainder indicated no such incident). This study indicated that although enacted stigma was relatively infrequent, felt stigma was common, and that both types were related to higher levels of distress.

Vardy et al. (2002) took this argument one step further, by using structural equation modelling to examine the link between disease severity, felt stigma and quality of life in patients with psoriasis. They showed that any link between disease severity and quality of life was completely mediated by expectations of stigmatisation. That is, severity of psoriasis had an impact on quality of life only insofar as it influenced expectations of being stigmatised by others.

Why does stigmatisation matter?

A fifth question concerns why stigmatisation has such a socially and personally significant effect on people. From a detached point of view, one might ask why experiences of the kinds illustrated above should have an impact but clearly they do. Simply reading the stigmatising experiences of other people often provokes an emotional response in the reader. Why is this so?

A very useful approach in this respect has been provided by Baumeister's (Baumeister & Tice, 1990; Leary, 1990) Social Exclusion Theory (SET). SET holds that a primary source of anxiety is potential exclusion from important social groups. It is based on three propositions that:

1 humans, as a species, possess a fundamental motive to avoid exclusion from social groupings;
2 much social behaviour reflects attempts to improve the chances of inclusion;
3 negative effect (including loneliness and depression) results when a person does not or cannot achieve a desired level of social inclusion.

In a recent set of experimental studies, Baumeister and colleagues (Baumeister et al., 2002; Sommer & Baumeister, 2002; Twenge et al., 2003) have demonstrated that the induction of beliefs about social exclusion and future loneliness can have a range of cognitive, emotional and behavioural consequences.

In a similar fashion, Hagerty and colleagues (Hagerty & Patusky, 1995; Hagerty et al., 1996; Hagerty & Williams, 1999) argue that the experience of personal involvement in a group, a sense of belonging, is a significant determinant of well-being. In their model, belonging has two attributes: being valued or needed by others and being congruent with others through shared characteristics. Depressed mood is a likely result when a sense of belonging is absent. Lee and Robbins (1995; 1998) have explored the role of social connectedness, defined as beliefs about enduring relationships with other people in general, rather than with particular individuals. It seems that stigmatisation matters to people because the rejection, or threat of rejection, taps into a fundamental human anxiety. Without good social connections, we are all more physically vulnerable.

How might stigmatisation be reduced?

A number of interventions have been developed to help people who are at risk of being stigmatised due to a difference in their appearance. Most have focused on the individual, but some have attempted to change societal attitudes and behaviour.

One approach is to reduce the visibility of a stigmatising mark. There is good evidence that cosmetic surgery (Sarwer et al., 1998) and cosmetic prostheses can help people feel better about themselves and their appearance. With respect to skin conditions, skin camouflage creams can be used to disguise skin blemishes such as scars and vitiligo. Kent (2002) found that clients who consulted the British Red Cross Skin Camouflage Service felt more confident in and exhibited less avoidance of social situations after their appointment than before. Although there was no measure of enacted or felt stigma in that study, qualitative comments indicated that clients were less preoccupied by how others would react to them. Laser treatment can also be helpful for those with port wine stains (Troilius et al., 1998), as is medical treatment for a variety of skin conditions including acne and eczema (Kurwa & Finlay, 1995; Kellett & Gawkrodger, 1999).

Other approaches are more psychologically based. Some aim to help people forestall stigmatisation. In social skills training people are encouraged to develop ways of displaying their social competence to others, so that the stigmatising condition is less pertinent to social interactions. Robinson et al. (1996) assessed the effects of a social skills workshop on the well-being of patients with a variety of disfiguring conditions. The package included instruction, modelling, role-play, feedback and discussion. Although there were improvements in levels of anxiety and social avoidance, again there were no measures of stigmatisation. Other approaches aim to help people to cope with stigmatisation when it occurs. Papadopoulous et al. (1999) used a cognitive–behavioural approach. They included an intervention intended to buffer the negative effects of stigmatisation by encouraging clients to engage in positive self-talk when anyone made a negative comment and to reframe staring as an indication of curiosity rather than rejection (Langer et al., 1976). They found a significant improvement in participants' quality of life, self-esteem and a decrease in negative automatic thoughts post-treatment, compared to a non-treatment comparison group.

However, these types of interventions concentrate on changing the appearance or the behaviour of the stigmatised individual, and do not address the wider issue of stigmatisation directly. The comparison would be with more recent approaches to physical disabilities; rather than locating problems of mobility with a person who uses a wheelchair, for example, it has become clear that there are central issues of physical access to the built environment. Just as changes in the physical environment can greatly reduce the disability of wheelchair use, changes in attitudes and behaviour of those who stigmatise could improve the well-being of those whose appearance is noticeably different.

People with visible differences sometimes take on this type of work themselves, seeking to inform others about the nature of their condition:

'Many years ago I went to a local swimming pool. After I had changed into my costume I entered the pool. As I walked toward the water I was approached by an attendant who asked what was wrong with my skin. He suggested that I shouldn't enter the water. I asked to see the manager and told him that his staff need better training'.

Unfortunately, there have been few formal attempts to make changes in these respects. Frances (2004) provides a detailed description of the interventions, supported by the UK charity *Changing Faces*, to assist children at school. Employing many of the same strategies that are used in anti-bullying programmes, Frances aims to develop school communities that are fully inclusive of children with visible differences. These interventions involve parents and teachers as well as children themselves. Cline et al. (1998) attempted to alter schoolchildren's attitudes and knowledge towards disfigurement by adding a theme into the school curriculum. Although the programme affected knowledge about and awareness of disfiguring conditions in the intervention schools as compared to control schools, there was no difference in the children's commitment to help others with disfigurements. There was no direct test of the effect of the intervention on behaviour.

Future research

This review suggests that there is scope for further research in a variety of areas, both personal (in terms of effects on individuals and the development of their coping skills) and social (in terms of understanding why stigmatisation occurs and how it might be reduced).

A number of studies reviewed above indicate that stigmatisation due to dermatological conditions can have far-reaching and long-term effects on individuals. However, almost all of this work has been cross-sectional. There is always the concern with this type of work that reports of stigmatisation, and their relationship to well-being, might only be due to response biases. That is, people who report low levels of self-esteem and high levels of distress might be vigilant for instances of stigmatisation and more likely to interpret 'neutral' events as instances of rejection. Indeed, Kent (1999) found that instances of enacted stigma were relatively uncommon, with reports of felt stigma being much more frequent. Respondents with vitiligo were much more likely to report that their skin condition affected their lives because of staring and the expectation of stigmatisation than stigmatisation itself. It would be very helpful in this respect to conduct some longitudinal work, perhaps by asking people to keep diaries of their experiences, so that the types of feelings, thoughts and behaviours of affected individuals could be charted more accurately.

Prospective studies could also be conducted. Given that stigmatising experiences seem so important to well-being and adjustment, regular interviews with people who have just begun to show symptoms of skin disease would be most informative. Although difficult to identify (given that most people have their symptoms for some time before seeking professional help, Thompson & Kent, 2001), following such a population would provide much information on the development of anxiety about appearance. In such studies it would be important to monitor feelings of shame and the use of concealment.

Such longitudinal and prospective studies could also provide data about coping strategies – how they are chosen, when they are used and whether they are successful in the short and longer term. Heason (2003) found that people with vitiligo tended to use a combination of problem-solving (e.g. telling others about the condition) and emotion-based (e.g. avoidance) coping strategies, but no information was collected about why and when a particular coping strategy was used. One could hypothesise that people who have experienced stigmatisation are more likely to use avoidance and concealment, a possibility open to testing.

However, it can be argued that the more important areas of research concern the reasons for stigmatisation and how it might be reduced. It would seem more practically useful, and perhaps more ethical given the paucity of resources devoted to helping people with dermatological conditions, to explore ways in which the frequency of stigmatisation can be changed. It may well be that, as Kurzban and Leary (2001) argue, there is a certain amount of hard wiring involved here. Beliefs could be operating out of consciousness and awareness. Reactions to skin diseases will be associated with neuronal activation in the brain. There is some work using functional magnetic resonance imaging (fMRI) to better understand a range of human emotions (Boguslawska et al., 1999), and it may be possible to identify the physiological processes relating to stigmatisation.

To the extent that people are stigmatised due to evolutionary pressures, rejection might be hard to reduce or forestall, especially when the perception of danger is involved. But, because there are cultural differences in the types of conditions that are stigmatised and because what is stigmatised changes over time, there must be a social component as well. Some degree of learning is involved; the question is how learning can be accomplished in a positive direction. Frances' (2004) case studies suggest that people can learn to overcome or reconsider attitudes towards those with disfigurements; the challenge is to explore how such changes can be accomplished on a wider, societal level.

REFERENCES

Albrecht, G.L., Walker, V., & Levy, J. (1982). Social distance from the stigmatized. A test of two theories. *Social Science and Medicine*, **16**, 1319–1327.

Bandura, A. (1977). *Social Learning Theory*, Englewood Cliffs, NJ: Prentice-Hall.

Baumeister, R., & Tice, D. (1990). Anxiety and social exclusion. *Journal of Social and Clinical Psychology*, **9**, 165–195.

Baumeister, R.F., Twenge, J.M., & Nuss, C.K. (2002). Effects of social exclusion on cognitive processes: anticipated aloneness reduces intelligent thought. *Journal of Personality and Social Psychology*, **83**, 817–827.

Boguslawska, R., Romanowski, C., Wilkinson, I., Montaldo, D., Singh, K., & Walecki, J. (1999). Introduction to functional magnetic resonance imaging. *Medical Science Monitor*, **5**, 1179–1186.

Cline, T., Proto, A., Raval, P., & Di Paolo, T. (1998). The effects of brief exposure and of classroom teaching on attitudes children express towards facial disfigurement in peers. *Educational Research*, **40**, 55–68.

Crandall, C., & Moriarty, D. (1995). Physical illness, stigma and social rejection. *Journal of Social Psychology*, **34**, 67–83.

Dion, K.K., Berscheid, E., & Walster, E. (1972). What is beautiful is good. *Journal of Personality and Social Psychology*, **24**, 285–290.

Eagly, A., Ashmore, R., Makhijani, M., & Longo, L. (1991). What is beautiful is good, but… A meta-analytic review of research on the physical attractiveness stereotype. *Psychological Bulletin*, **110**, 109–128.

Finlay, A., & Khan, G. (1994). Dermatology life quality index (DLQI): a simple practical measure for routine clinical use. *Clinical and Experimental Dermatology*, **19**, 210–216.

Frances, J. (2004). *Educating Children with Facial Disfigurement: Creating Inclusive School Communities*. London: Routledge Falmer.

Gilbert, P. (2000). What is shame? In: P. Gilbert, & B. Andrews (Eds), *Shame: Interpersonal Behaviour, Psychopathology and Culture* (pp. 3–37). New York: Oxford University Press.

Ginsburg, I., & Link, B. (1989). Feelings of stigmatization in patients with psoriasis. *Journal of the American Academy of Dermatology*, **20**, 53–63.

Goffman, E. (1968). *Stigma*. London: Penguin.

Gupta, M., Gupta, A., & Watteel, G. (1998). Perceived deprivation of social touch in psoriasis is associated with greater psychological morbidity: an index of the stigma experience in dermatologic disorders. *Cutis*, **61**, 339–342.

Hagerty, B.M.K., & Patusky, K. (1995). Developing a measure of sense of belonging. *Nursing Research*, **44**, 9–13.

Hagerty, B.M., & Williams, R.A. (1999). The effects of sense of belonging, social support, conflict, and loneliness on depression. *Nursing Research*, **48**, 215–219.

Hagerty, B.M., Williams, R.A., Coyne, J.C., & Early, M.R. (1996). Sense of belonging and indicators of social and psychological functioning. *Archives of Psychiatric Nursing*, **10**, 235–244.

Heason, S.L. (2003). *The Development of a Model of Disfigurement: The Process of Living with Vitiligo*. Sheffield: Unpublished PhD Thesis, University of Sheffield.

Heatherton, T.F., Kleck, R.E., Hebl, M.R. & Hull, J.G. (2000). *The Social Psychology of Stigma*. New York: Guildford.

Houston, B., & Bull, R. (1994). Do people avoid sitting next to someone who is facially disfigured? *European Journal of Social Psychology*, **24**, 279–284.

Jacoby, A. (1994). Felt versus enacted stigma: a concept revisited. *Social Science and Medicine*, **38**, 269–274.

Jones, E., Farina, A., Hastorf, A., Markus, H., Miller, D., & Scott, R. (1984). *Social Stigma. The Psychology of Marked Relationships*. New York: Freeman.

Kellett, S., & Gawkrodger, D. (1999). The psychological and emotional impact of acne and the effect of treatment with isotretinoin. *British Journal of Dermatology*, **140**, 273–282.

Kent, G. (1999). Correlates of perceived stigma in vitiligo. *Psychology & Health*, **14**, 241–252.

Kent, G. (2002). Testing a model of disfigurement: effects of a skin camouflage service on well-being and appearance anxiety. *Psychology & Health*, **17**, 377–386.

Kent, G., & Keohane, S. (2001). Social anxiety and disfigurement: the moderating effects of fear of negative evaluation and past experience. *British Journal of Clinical Psychology*, **40**, 23–34.

Kleck, R., & Strenta, A. (1980). Perceptions of the impact of negatively valued physical characteristics on social interaction. *Journal of Personality and Social Psychology*, **39**, 861–873.

Kurwa, H., & Finlay, A. (1995). Dermatology in-patient management greatly improves quality of life. *British Journal of Dermatology*, **133**, 575–578.

Kurzban, R., & Leary, M. (2001). Evolutionary origins of stigmatization: the functions of social exclusion. *Psychological Bulletin*, **127**, 187–208.

Langer, E., Fiske, S., Taylor, S., & Chanowitz, B. (1976). Stigma, staring, and discomfort: a novel-stimulus hypothesis. *Journal of Experimental and Social Psychology*, **12**, 451–463.

Leary, M. (1990). Responses to social exclusion: social anxiety, jealousy, loneliness, depression, and low self-esteem. *Journal of Social and Clinical Psychology*, **9**, 221–229.

Lee, R.M., & Robbins, S.B. (1995). Measuring belongingness – the social connectedness and the social assurance scales. *Journal of Counseling Psychology*, **42**, 232–241.

Lee, R.M., & Robbins, S.B. (1998). The relationship between social connectedness and anxiety, self-esteem, and social identity. *Journal of Counseling Psychology*, **45**, 338–345.

Lerner, M., & Miller, D. (1978). Just world research and the attribution process: looking back and ahead. *Psychological Bulletin*, **85**, 1030–1051.

Martini, T., & Page, S. (1998). Attributions and the stigma of illiteracy: understanding help seeking in low literate adults. *Canadian Journal of Behavioural Science*, **28**, 121–129.

Papadopoulous, L., Bor, R., & Legg, C. (1999). Coping with the disfiguring effects of vitiligo: a preliminary investigation into the effects of cognitive behavioural therapy. *British Journal of Medical Psychology*, **10**, 11–12.

Rapp, S., Feldman, S., Exum, M., Fleischer, A., & Reboussin, D. (1999). Psoriasis causes as much disability as other major medical diseases. *Journal of the American Academy of Dermatology*, **41**, 401–407.

Robinson, E., Rumsey, N., & Partidge, J. (1996). An evaluation of the impact of social interaction skills training for facially disfigured people. *British Journal of Plastic Surgery*, **49**, 281–289.

Rozin, P., & Fallon, A. (1987). A perspective on disgust. *Psychological Review*, **94**, 23–41.

Rumsey, N., Bull, R., & Gahagan, D. (1982). The effect of facial disfigurement on the proxemic behaviour of the general public. *Journal of Applied Social Psychology*, **12**, 137–150.

Sarwer, D., Wadden, T., Pertchuk, M., & Whitaker, L. (1998). The psychology of cosmetic surgery: a review and reconceptualization. *Clinical Psychology Review*, **18**, 1–22.

Schmid-Ott, G., Jaeger, B., Kuensebeck, H., Ott, R., & Lamprecht, F. (1996). Dimensions of stigmatisation in patients with psoriasis in a questionnaire on experience with skin complaints. *Dermatology*, **193**, 304–310.

Smart, L., & Wegner, D. (1999). Covering up what can't be seen: concealable stigma and mental control. *Journal of Personality and Social Psychology*, **77**, 474–486.

Sommer, K.L., & Baumeister, R.F. (2002). Self-evaluation, persistence, and performance following implicit rejection: the role of trait self-esteem. *Personality and Social Psychology Bulletin*, **28**, 926–938.

Thompson, A., & Kent, G. (2001). Adjusting to disfigurement: processes involved in dealing with being visibly different. *Clinical Psychology Review*, **21**, 663–682.

Troilius, A., Wrangsjo, B., & Ljunggren, B. (1998). Potential psychological benefits from early treatment of port-wine stains in children. *British Journal of Dermatology*, **139**, 59–65.

Twenge, J.M., Catanese, K.R., & Baumeister, R.F. (2003). Social exclusion and the deconstructed state: time perception, meaninglessness, lethargy, lack of emotion, and self-awareness. *Journal of Personality and Social Psychology*, **85**, 409–423.

Vardy, D., Besser, A., Amir, M., Gesthalter, B., Biton, A., & Buskila, D. (2002). Experiences of stigmatization play a role in mediating the impact of disease severity on quality of life in psoriasis patients. *British Journal of Dermatology*, **147**, 736–742.

Wahl, A.K., Gjengedal, E., & Hanestad, B.R. (2002). The bodily suffering of living with severe psoriasis: in depth interviews with 22 hospitalised patients with psoriasis. *Qualitative Health Research*, **12**, 250–261.

Weiner, B., Perry, R., & Magnusson, J. (1988). An attributional analysis of reactions to stigmas. *Journal of Personality and Social Psychology*, **55**, 738–748.

5

Coping with chronic skin conditions: factors important in explaining individual variation in adjustment

Andrew Thompson

Introduction

It is increasingly acknowledged that whilst it is likely that a large number of people living with skin conditions adjust well to their condition, there is a risk for some of them experiencing social, psychological, and physical distress (Gupta, Chapter 3, this volume). In common with other chronic illnesses and appearance-altering conditions there appears to be no simple relationship between single biomedical and demographical factors, such as severity and age, and psychological adjustment (Papadopoulos et al., 1999a; Thompson & Kent, 2001; Rumsey & Harcourt, 2004).

This chapter reviews the literature pertaining to adjusting to a life with a chronic dermatological condition. It aims to briefly outline the potential psychosocial impacts and then detail the likely factors that have been implicated in playing key mediating roles in explaining individual variation in coping and adjustment.

Defining 'skin conditions'

Consideration of dermatological diagnoses is outside of the remit of this chapter and those interested are referred to an appropriate medical text (e.g. Gawkrodger, 2002). However, it is important to acknowledge that there are multiple types of skin conditions, which can differ widely in terms of both specific symptoms and treatments, as such factors may have an impact upon the adjustment process (Porter et al., 1986). The term 'skin condition' as opposed to skin disease, will be used here when discussing this population in general, so as to be inclusive of the full range of dermatological conditions. This will include those acquired congenitally, such as port wine stains, as well as those resulting from diseases, such as psoriasis.

What do people living with chronic skin conditions have to cope with?

Living with the ongoing stressors associated with any chronic condition generally requires the development of skills to regain a sense of equilibrium (Moos & Schaefer, 1984). Unfortunately, for people living with chronic skin conditions, as well as the physical symptoms there are often a range of treatment, psychological and social issues associated with it that can act as stressors in their own right (Papadopoulos et al., 1999a). The potential impact of such issues will now be briefly addressed.

The symptoms and their treatments

Certainly, the physical symptoms associated with specific conditions can cause, amongst other things, pain, irritation, and disability, as the following quote highlights:

'The only place I get any relief is in the bath, 20 minutes a time, then itch, itch, itch, red blotches everywhere.' ('Evidence' submitted by a woman living with eczema to the All Party Parliamentary Group on Skin (2003, p. 4))

In addition, treatments can involve the use of messy and/or unpleasant smelling creams, such as coal tar-based ointments and camouflaging cosmetics, and regular attendance at clinics for time-consuming therapies, such as ultraviolet (UV) A\B light therapy (Miles, 2002). The following quotes testify to these difficulties:

'I don't want to go through all this rigmarole every day, putting this stuff (camouflage and sun-block) on.'
                    Quote from a woman with vitiligo cited in Thompson et al. (2002, p. 219)

'Smearing on the evil-smelling, sticky, staining stuff could take up to two or more hours a day, soaking in it another hour or so. Visits to the clinic absorbed another five or six hours a week.' ('Evidence' submitted by a man living with psoriasis to the All Party Parliamentary Group on Skin (2003, p. 5))

Further, medications developed for use with dermatological treatment can also have dangerous side effects, which can include triggering psychiatric symptoms, and for this reason they often require careful monitoring. For example, isotretinoin used in the treatment of acne has been linked to depression (Kellett & Gawkrodger, 1999; Ng & Schweitzer, 2003) and Dapsone, another dermatological medication, has been linked to manic-depression (Gawkrodger, 1989; Zhu & Stiller, 2001).

The social and psychological impact of skin conditions

To some extent skin conditions are unique from many other diseases in so far as they are often visible to others, and as a result social factors associated with both appearance and illness are relevant to the adjustment process. There is no doubt that living with a chronic skin condition can be stigmatising (Kent, Chapter 4, this volume). As early as 1976 Jobling found that for psoriasis sufferers the greatest psychosocial impact of having the condition were interpersonal difficulties. It is now widely established that individuals with a disfiguring skin condition can suffer negative and intrusive reactions from others as well as experiencing interpersonal difficulties, such as in the formation of relationships (e.g. Jowett & Ryan, 1985; Lanigan & Cotterill, 1989). The following quote typifies the simple intrusive reactions that people living with a skin condition can experience:

'I mean it does get you sometimes. If you see them actually staring at you'. (Quote from a woman with vitiligo cited in Thompson et al. (2002, p. 219))

Studies using confederates made up to look as if they had some form of facial blemish, such as a birth-mark, have found that people tend to be less helpful, less charitable, and offer less sympathy to people with a disfigurement across a range of settings (Samerotte & Harris, 1976; Bull & Stevens, 1981; Rumsey et al., 1982; Kerr et al., 1985). Indeed there is emerging evidence that people hold negative implicit attitudes (attitudes that have not been subject to modification in response to factors, such as social desirability) towards people with visible skin conditions (Grandfield et al., 2004).

Although the tendency of others to react negatively towards people with visible skin conditions is well established, relatively little theoretical or experimental consideration has been given to exploring the causes of this phenomenon. Hypotheses to account for these reactions have revolved around evolutionary theory (Kellett & Gilbert, 2001; Thompson & Kent, 2001), fear and uncertainty (Partridge, 1996) and primitive beliefs often linked to concepts of 'fate' or a 'just world' (Shaw, 1981). Certainly, a whole collection of negative, culturally bound, beliefs relating to skin conditions exist, often related to the occurrence and maintenance of the condition as relating to personality flaws in the sufferer. For example, Alderman (1989) has described a collection of 'acne myths' relating to such ideas as acne being caused by poor diet and hygiene. Beuf (1990) has reported a belief amongst the Black American population, that the depigmenting condition vitiligo occurs as a punishment for harbouring hidden desires to be white.

Further research is needed to explore the degree to which such stigma relates to stereotypes or that evolutionary predisposed mechanisms are linked to avoiding contamination and maintaining rank, although it is likely that both are involved (Thompson & Kent, 2001). However, what is clear is that such an 'ongoing sociocultural' context forms an additional stressor for those living with skin condition to have to cope with. This context may also be instrumental in the formation of an individuals' own representations/beliefs concerning their condition and the values they attribute to appearance generally, and as such is likely to be crucially implicated in adjustment. The role of such cognitive factors will be discussed later.

Perhaps not surprisingly given the potential, social, and physical consequences previously described, elevated levels of psychological morbidity have been reported within the literature (Harlow et al., 2000; Picardi et al., 2001; Picardi et al., 2003a). The kind of psychological difficulties commonly found have included: anxiety (e.g. Jowett & Ryan, 1985); depression including risk of suicide (e.g. Hughes et al., 1983; Cotterill & Cunliffe, 1997; Humphreys & Humphreys, 1998); lowered self-esteem (e.g. Jowett & Ryan, 1985; Porter & Beuf, 1988; Van der Donk et al., 1994); feelings of shame (e.g. Jowett & Ryan, 1985; Salzer & Schallreuter, 1995; Thompson et al., 2002); and concerns with body image (e.g. Papadopoulos et al., 1999b; Benrud-Larson et al., 2003).

Indeed, the association between self-concept and appearance is supported by a range of studies (Thompson & Kent, 2001) and there are vivid qualitative accounts of the potential impact on the overall self-concept provided within the literature as the following quote demonstrates:

'No matter what the objective reality, in my heart I think of myself as I was in my teens. I will always be a freak, someone deeply unworthy, someone lurking on the fringes of humanity.' (Richardson, 1997, p. 61)

Individual variation in the psychosocial impact

Whilst the literature indicates that there are generally higher levels of psychological distress amongst people with skin conditions, there is also evidence to suggest that there is considerable individual variation. Indeed, several studies have found that the psychosocial impact of living with a chronic skin condition can be minimal. For example, Kalick et al. (1981) in their study of individuals living with a port wine stain seeking laser therapy, found no evidence of heightened levels of distress. Ben-Tovim and Walker (1995) studied body-related attitudes in a small sample of women with a range of disfiguring dermatological conditions and found that the women did not disparage their bodies to a greater extent than a matched control group.

The 'Holy Grail' of both chronic illness and disfigurement research is to account for the variation in individual distress and to identify the key factors that are involved in adjustment, thus allowing the development of appropriate psychosocial interventions. The identification of such factors is perhaps even more important in skin conditions given the role they may play in exacerbating the actual physical condition itself (Millard, Chapter 2, this volume).

Explanatory factors in coping and adjustment

Research on this topic can be grouped into five themes: disease and treatment factors; predisposing developmental factors; ongoing sociocultural factors; cognitive/

Early experiences and cultural stereotypes (predisposing developmental factors)
Values placed on appearance and skin by family and society
Stereotypes connected with specific conditions
Actual early experiences of being accepted or rejected

↓

Disease and treatment factors
Specific disease/condition. Visibility. Age of onset. Severity. Nature of treatments

↓↑

Cognitive factors: Personality characteristics and core beliefs
Personality characteristics (i.e. alexithymia, shame proneness, and attachment styles)
Appearance schemas and self-discrepancies. Illness representations
(i.e. personal beliefs about the specific illness)

↓↑

Feelings/distress related to skin condition

↓↑

Coping strategies
Interpersonal/social skills. Emotion focused and problem focused coping

↓↑

Ongoing sociocultural factors
Social support (acceptance) versus social rejection (discrimination,
prejudice, negative stereotypes, and automatic reactions)

Figure 5.1   Model of the interacting factors implicated in the origin and maintenance of skin-specific affect/distress.

personality factors; and coping style factors. These factors are summarised and represented schematically in Figure 5.1.

Disease and treatment factors

As previously stated, the literature suggests that objective factors, such as age of onset, severity, type of skin condition and type of treatment received, are only weak or poor predictors of adjustment. Whilst, qualitative accounts clearly testify to the potential for treatments to be predictive factors related to distress, there have been few studies that have actually looked at this with any sufficient rigour. Indeed, there is some evidence to suggest that treatment factors are not significantly associated with disability or quality of life (Fortune et al., 1997).

Numerous studies have found only a weak association between disease severity and psychological functioning (Finlay et al., 1990; Clark et al., 1997; Fortune et al., 1997; Fortune et al., 2002). Clinician and self-report measures of severity generally do not correlate, nor do clinical ratings of severity and measures of disability. Whilst, Finlay et al. (1990) found a moderate correlation between clinically measured severity and disability (as measured by the Psoriasis Disability Index (PDI)), the majority of other studies have not found such a relationship. For example, Root et al. (1994) also used the PDI in their study of psoriasis and found that there was not a correlation between clinician-rated severity, and distress or disability. However, they found that there were 'moderately high' correlations between self-rated severity and disability and distress. Their analyses further suggested that the relationship between self-rated severity and distress was mediated by disability. They consequently concluded that self-rated severity was associated with social avoidance, which in turn was related to psychological distress. However, the problem with many of the studies that have looked at self-rated severity is that they have largely failed to define what severity means to the sufferer and it maybe that severity, disability and distress are perceived synonymously.

Given the stigmatising reactions of others, it could be expected that increased visibility would be associated with heightened levels of psychological distress. There is some evidence for this but even here the findings are equivocal. Hughes et al. (1983) found that 70% of their sample with visible skin conditions had heightened the levels of psychological distress. Picardi et al. (2001) found that visibility was an important predictive factor for psychological distress for women. However, Fortune et al. (1997) in their study of psoriasis sufferers found only a modest association.

Whilst, the potential for heightened levels of psychological distress have been found across the range of chronic skin conditions, there is some evidence that there may be differences between specific conditions. Porter et al. (1986) reported poorer adjustment amongst their participants with psoriasis as opposed to those with vitiligo, although both groups experienced lower self-esteem than a control group. Interestingly, the people with psoriasis also reported experiencing more negative reactions from others than the vitiligo group. Type of condition is often also associated with age of onset, insofar as some conditions are congenital whilst others are typically acquired in adolescence and others later in life. This makes it difficult to disentangle disease-specific factors from developmental factors. Again the literature relating to age of onset is also somewhat equivocal. For example, although Porter and Beuf (1988) found a difference between age groups amongst people living with vitiligo, they reported that there was much variation within their age groups, suggesting factors other than age are important. It seems likely that the relationship between disability, distress and disease-related factors is likely to be mediated by other 'higher order' factors, which will be discussed below.

Predisposing developmental factors

The birth of a child with a disfiguring skin condition can be very stressful or at least a shock for parents. Langlois and Sawin (1981) found that 2-day-old infants judged to be less attractive were held less close and given less attention than infants judged to be attractive. Such early reactions may disturb attachments, predisposing a child to the later development of psychological distress. Although it is likely that the majority of parents quickly overcome any initial negative reactions, some may continue to struggle to truly accept their child (Walters, 1997; Kent & Thompson, 2002; Rumsey & Harcourt, 2004).

In addition, we live in a society where a premium is placed on appearance and, as stated earlier, the reactions of others to those with a noticeable disfigurement can be less than charitable. Other children can be particularly discriminatory and those children with an altered appearance can be singled out for bullying and social exclusion. Typically, we face constant messages from the media that to be beautiful is also to be good (Dion et al., 1972). Indeed, children's stories often carry the message that to be disfigured or different in appearance is to be bad in some way (*'Out popped the troll's ugly head. He was so ugly that the youngest Billy-goat Gruff nearly fell down with fright': The Three Billy Goats Gruff*; cited in Kent & Thompson, 2002).

As previously stated, children are likely to internalise the prevalent stereotypes and any consistent negative reactions received from others, particularly significant others. Such factors are likely to be instrumental in shaping underlying cognitive structures associated with self-concept and personality. Indeed, Cash and Labarge (1996), and Altabe and Thompson (1996) have defined body image in terms of appearance-related schemas or mental representations developed in childhood.

Ongoing sociocultural factors

Acquiring a skin condition in later life can also be distressing and attract negative reactions from others. Adolescence is a particularly sensitive time for the development of self-concept (see Richardson, 1997, above). Experiencing distress on acquiring a skin condition later in life has been hypothesised (Kent & Thompson, 2002) to be related to either the confirmation of existing predisposing underlying negative beliefs, or to discrepancies arising between existing positive self-beliefs and actual self, as predicted by self-discrepancy theory (Higgins, 1987). As such, the personal value (appearance schemas) one previously attributed to one's appearance may be a critical factor for some in dictating the degree of discrepancy and the consequential distress experienced.

Clearly then, feeling accepted by significant others maybe crucial to psychological well-being at any time in life. Cobb (1976) has defined social support as information leading people to believe that they are valued by others. Social support may serve to facilitate a sense of being accepted (Thompson & Kent, 2002). This may partly explain why social support has emerged as being linked to adjustment (Kalick et al., 1981; Picardi et al., 2003b, d).

Cognitive factors: personality characteristics and core beliefs

Predisposing developmental factors are clearly linked to the development of several personality characteristics that are emerging as having predictive power in explaining some of the variability in adjustment. Whilst disrupted attachments in childhood have been discussed as having the potential to lead to stable attachment styles in adulthood, few studies have actually explored the role of attachment, and those that have, were unable to relate this directly back to early experiences. Picardi et al. (2003b, c, d) found higher levels of insecure and avoidant attachment styles in a small sample of people with newly diagnosed or recently exacerbated vitiligo and alopecia areata. Interestingly, their participants also had poorer levels of social support and it was hypothesised that this might result from difficulties in accessing social support as a result of the underlying attachment style.

Shame-proneness is another personality factor linked to early relationships (Tangey & Fischer, 1995; Gilbert & Miles, 2002). Feelings of shame have frequently been described by some people living with chronic skin conditions (e.g. Jowett & Ryan, 1985). Indeed, it has been argued that shame, self-esteem, appearance consciousness, fear of negative evaluation, and social anxiety are all similar concepts, in terms of their developmental origins, their relation to one's sense of being accepted by others, and their underlying cognitive processes (Thompson, 1998). This may explain why some earlier studies have found self-esteem to be closely related to adjustment (Porter et al., 1990; Van der Donk et al., 1994).

Further support to the important role played by these overlapping concepts is provided by the findings of Fortune et al. (1997) with a group of people living with psoriasis. Whilst, they found only a modest association between visibility and distress, their analyses revealed that stress resulting from anticipating negative reactions from others accounted for more of the variance in disability scores than any other disease-related factor. This finding is lent further support by qualitative research which suggests 'social vulnerability' is a key concern for those living with a skin condition (Thompson et al., 2002; Wahl et al., 2002). Further, quantitative evidence is provided by Leary et al. (1998) and Kent and Keohane (2001) who made use of the Brief Fear of Negative Evaluation Scale (FNE: Leary, 1983) and found that this conceptually-related factor moderated the degree of distress experienced. Papadopoulos et al. (1999b) and Kent (2002) have also found heightened levels of appearance-related negative thoughts and beliefs, respectively in samples of vitiligo and camouflage service users.

Two other cognitive factors have recently attracted attention in this area, alexithymia and illness representations. Alexithymia has been described as a set of stable personality difficulties related to moderating affect. Alexithymics are described as having difficulty with both emotional expression and experiencing, and possibly have heightened sensitivity to anxiety. Such traits may impact negatively on physical health via heightening physiological arousal to misperceived threats (Kauhanen et al., 1994; Fortune et al., 2002). Elevated levels of alexithymia have recently been reported amongst people with vitiligo (Picardi et al., 2003b), psoriasis (Allegranti et al., 1994; Fortune et al., 2002; Picardi et al., 2003c), and alopecia areata (Picardi et al., 2003d). Fortune et al. (2002) found that people with psoriasis who scored highly on a measure of alexithymia also scored highly on a measure of anxiety, even after illness perceptions and coping factors (which will be discussed below) were accounted for. Alexithymia was also associated, although to a lesser extent, with higher depression, stress and worrying, but not with higher disability.

As already stated, beliefs concerning illness development are likely to be important factors in adjustment. Leventhal et al. (1980, 1992) have developed a model of illness representations to define key areas of common sense beliefs that appear important in adjustment to chronic illness. Illness representations are concerned with causal attributions, perceived consequences, beliefs associated with control and treatment, duration, and illness identity (symptom perception). As previously stated, lay beliefs about the origin and maintenance of skin conditions abound and may differ across cultures. Beliefs within the illness representation domains have been shown to be influential in medical help-seeking. Scharloo et al. (2000) found that people with psoriasis made greater use of outpatient services if they believed that their condition had serious consequences, was controllable, and they had a heightened illness identity. Fortune et al. (2002) have reported that illness perceptions were the most useful variables (in comparison to coping factors and alexithymia, which were also important) in accounting for psoriasis-related distress, stress and disability. Further, Fortune et al. (2004) have shown that such beliefs are amenable to psychosocial intervention.

Clearly, these cognitive personality factors warrant further study in order to examine their role in interventions. In addition, clarification is needed as to whether they actually do represent underlying stable personality traits or whether they are best thought of as situationally applied coping mechanisms. However, what is clear is that they are related to and possibly instrumental in the types of coping strategies deployed.

Coping

Coping refers to the many strategies (cognitive, behavioural and emotional) used to manage specific stressors. Lazurus and Folkman's (1984) transactional model is currently the predominant model of coping. This model suggests that through a process of primary and secondary appraisal, an individual will make use of a range of coping strategies. The available range can be broadly split into those that are aimed either at directly tackling the stressor itself, so-called problem-focused strategies (e.g. confronting someone who is staring), or those that are aimed at regulating the emotional impact, so-called emotion-focused strategies (e.g. denial). A simplified picture is that situations that can become controlled are best dealt with by the former strategies, whilst those that are not changeable are best addressed by emotion-focused strategies.

All of the personality and cognitive factors described above have clear links to the types of coping strategies deployed by individuals. Shame-proneness, alexithymia, and avoidant-attachment style have all been linked to avoidant-coping strategies. For example, vitiligo and alopecia areata participants with higher levels of insecure and avoidant-attachment styles also had poorer levels of social support and it was hypothesised that this might result from difficulties in being able to access social support (Picardi et al., 2003b, c, d).

Avoidance, concealment, escape, and the use of subtle safety behaviours (such as turning one's body so as to hide one's perceived worse side in social situations) are all common shame and social anxiety-related coping strategies. Such coping mechanisms have frequently been linked to poor adjustment (Rapp et al., 2001; Hill & Kennedy, 2002; Kent, 2002). However, this picture is not clear cut, in so much as people may recognise the limitations of using such strategies and feel ambivalent in their use of them, but nevertheless feel recourse to do so as other strategies (such as being socially proactive) may be more demanding of personal resources (Thompson, 1998). Nevertheless, coping factors are clearly important in accounting for differences in adjustment and warrant further study. Importantly, there is growing evidence that interventions aimed at helping people to develop coping skills to manage the reactions of other can be useful (Robinson et al., 1996).

Conclusion

A significant problem in estimating the true impact and role of psychosocial factors in this area relates to the fact that the studies conducted have largely been based on unrepresentative samples drawn either from hospital clinics or self-help organisations. Such groups may not be representative of the whole population of people affected and probably contain people whose conditions are more severe, in early onset, or that have had a greater impact upon them. Clearly, more research needs to be conducted within community and primary care settings in order to replicate and enhance the findings described above.

This chapter makes the case for adjustment being seen as a complex, multifaceted, and ongoing biopsychosocial process, operating not only at the level of the individual with the condition but also at a societal level. Indeed, encountering negative reactions of others maybe unavoidable (Grandfield et al., 2004), although clearly individual differences in adjustment seem undoubtedly linked to the ways people think and in turn react to both internal and external threats. It is likely that complex interactions between underlying cognitive factors (such as shame-proneness) and social reactions are largely responsible for mediating the nature of coping and in turn the degree of distress and disability experienced. Research has only just begun to examine the roles of such factors in the implementation of psychosocial interventions and further research is needed here.

REFERENCES

Alderman, C. (1989). Not just skin deep. *Nursing Standard*, **37**, 22–24.

Allegranti, I., Gon, T., Magaton-Rizzi, G., & Aguglia, E. (1994). Prevalence of alexithymia characteristics in psoriatic patients. *Acta Dermatologica Vererologica*, **186**, 146–147.

All Party Parliamentary Group on Skin (2003). *Report on the enquiry into the impact of skin diseases on people's lives*. London: HMSO.

Altabe, M., & Thompson, J.K., (1996). Body image: a cognitive self-schema construct. *Cognitive Therapy and Research*, **20**, 171–193.

Benrud-Larson, L.M., Heinberg, L.J., Boling, C., Reed, J., White, B., Wigley, F.M., & Haythornwaite, J.A. (2003). Body image dissatisfaction among women with scleroderma: extent and relationship to psychosocial function. *Health Psychology*, **22**, 130–139.

Ben-Tovim, D., & Walker, M.K. (1995). Body image, disfigurement and disability. *Journal of Psychosomatic Research*, **39**, 283–291.

Beuf, A. (1990). *Beauty is the Beast*. Philadelphia: University of Pennsylvania Press.

Bull, R., & Stevens, J. (1981). The effects of facial disfigurement on helping behaviour. *The Italian Journal of Psychology*, **8**, 25–31.

Cash, T.F., & Labarge, A.S. (1996). Development of the appearance schemas inventory: a new cognitive body-image assessment. *Cognitive Therapy and Research*, **20**, 37–50.

Cotterill, J.A., & Cunliffe, W.J. (1997). Suicide in dermatology patients. *British Journal of Dermatology*, **137**, 246–250.

Clark, S.M., Goulden, V., Finlay, A.Y., & Cunliffe, W.J. (1997). The psychological and social impact of acne: a comparison study using 3 acne disability questionnaires. *British Journal of Dermatology Supplement*, **137**, 41–42.

Cobb, S. (1976). Social support as a moderator of life stress. *Psychosomatic Medicine*, **38**, 300–314.

Dion, K.K., Berscheid, E., & Walster, E. (1972). What is beautiful is good. *Journal of Personality and Social Psychology*, **11**, 1–18.

Finlay, A.Y., Khan, G.K., Luscombe, D.K., & Salek, M.S. (1990). Validation of sickness impact profile and psoriasis disability index in psoriasis. *British Journal of Dermatology*, **123**, 751–756.

Fortune, D.G., Main, C.J., O'Sullivan, T.M., & Griffiths, C.E.M. (1997). Quality of life in patients with psoriasis: the contribution of clinical variables and psoriasis-specific stress. *British Journal of Dermatology*, **137**, 755–760.

Fortune, D.G., Richards, H.L., Griffiths, E.M., & Main, C. (2002). Psychological stress, distress and disability in patients with psoriasis: consensus and variation in the contribution of illness perceptions, coping and alexithymia. *British Journal of Clinical Psychology*, **41**, 157–174.

Fortune, D.G., Richards, H.L., Griffiths, C.E.M., & Main, C.J. (2004). Targeting cognitive-behaviour therapy to patients' implicit model of psoriasis: results from a patient preference controlled trial. *British Journal of Clinical Psychology*, **43**, 65–82.

Gawkrodger, D. (1989). Manic depression induced by dapsone in patient with dermatitis-herpetiformis. *British Medical Journal*, **299(6703)**, 860.

Gawkrodger, D.J. (2002). *Dermatology: An Illustrated Colour Text*, 3rd edn. Edinburgh: Churchill Livingstone.

Gilbert, P., & Miles, J. (2002). *Body Shame: Conceptualization, Research and Treatment*. Hove: Bruner-Routledge.

Grandfield, T., Thompson, A., & Turpin, G. (2004). An attitudinal study of responses to dermatitis using the implicit association test. Poster presented at the *Annual British Psychological Society Conference*, April.

Harlow, D., Poyner, T., Finlay, A.Y., & Dykes, P.J. (2000). Impaired quality of life of adults with skin disease in primary care. *British Journal of Dermatology*, **143**, 979–982.

Hill, L., & Kennedy, P. (2002). The role of coping strategies in mediating subjective disability in people who have psoriasis. *Psychology, Health and Medicine*, **7**, 261–269.

Higgins, E. (1987). Self-discrepancy: a theory relating to self and affect. *Psychological Review*, **94**, 319–340.

Hughes, J., Barraclough, B., Hamblin, L., & White, J. (1983). Psychiatric symptoms in dermatology patients. *British Journal of Psychiatry*, **143**, 51–54.

Humphreys, S., & Humphreys, R. (1998). Psychiatric morbidity and skin disease: what dermatologists think they see. *British Journal of Dermatology*, **139**, 679–681.

Jobling, R. (1976). Psoriasis: a preliminary questionnaire study of sufferers' subjective experience. *Clinical and Experimental Dermatology*, **1**, 233.

Jowett, S., & Ryan, T. (1985). Skin disease and handicap: an analysis of the impact of skin conditions. *Social Science and Medicine*, **20**, 424–429.

Kalick, S., Goldwyn, R., & Noe, J. (1981). Social issues and body image concerns of port wine stain patients undergoing laser therapy. *Lasers in Surgery and Medicine*, **1**, 205–213.

Kauhanen, J., Kaplan, G.A., Julkunen, J., & Salonen, J.T. (1994). The association of alexithymia with all cause mortality: prospective epidemiologic evidence. *Psychosomatic Medicine*, **56**, 149.

Kellett, S.C., & Gawkroger, D.J. (1999). The psychological and emotional impact of acne and the effect of treatment with isotretinoin. *British Journal of Dermatology*, **140**, 273–282.

Kellett, S., & Gilbert, P. (2001). Acne: a biopsychosocial and evolutionary perspective with a focus on shame. *British Journal of Health Psychology*, **6**, 1–24.

Kent, G. (2002). Testing a model of disfigurement: effects of a skin camouflage service on well being and appearance anxiety. *Psychology and Health*, **17**, 377–386.

Kent, G., & Keohane, S. (2001). Social anxiety and disfigurement: the moderating effects of fear of negative evaluation and past experience. *British Journal of Clinical Psychology*, **40**, 339–342.

Kent, G., & Thompson, A. (2002). The development and maintenance of shame in disfigurement. In: P. Gilbert & L. Miles (Eds), *Body Shame: Conceptualisation, Research and Treatment*, New York: Brunner-Routledge.

Kerr, R.L., Bull, R.H.C., MacCoun, R.J., & Rathborn, H. (1985). Judgements of victim attractiveness, care and disfigurement on the judgements of American and British mock jurors. *Journal of Social Psychology*, **24**, 47–58.

Langlois, J., & Sawin, D. (1981). Infant physical attractiveness as an elicitor of differential parenting behaviours. Paper presented at the Society for Research in Child Development, Boston. Cited in Walters, E. (1997). Problems faced by children and families living with visible differences. In: R. Lansdown, N. Rumsey, E. Bradbury, T. Carr, & J. Partridge (Eds), *Visibly Different: Coping with Disfigurement*. Oxford: Butterworth-Heinemann.

Lanigan, S., & Cotterill, J. (1989). Psychological disabilities amongst patients with port wine stains. *British Journal of Dermatology*, **121**, 209–215.

Lazurus, R., & Folkman, S. (1984). *Stress, Appraisal and Coping*. New York: Springer.

Leary, M. (1983). A brief version of the fear of negative evaluation scale. *Personality and Social Psychology Bulletin*, **9**, 371–376.

Leary, M., Rapp, S., Herbst, K., Exum, M., & Feldman, S. (1998). Interpersonal concerns and psychological difficulties of psoriasis patients: effects of disease severity and fear of negative evaluation. *Health Psychology*, **17**, 1–7.

Leventhal, H., Diefenbach, M., & Leventhal, E. (1992). Illness cognition: using common sense to understand treatment adherence and affect cognition interactions. *Cognitive Therapy and Research*, **16**, 143–163.

Leventhal, H., Meyer, D., & Nerenz, D. (1980). The common sense representation of illness danger. In: S. Rachman (Ed.), *Contributions to Medical Psychology* (Vol. 2.), New York: Pergamon Press, pp. 7–30.

Miles, J. (2002). Psoriasis: The role of shame on quality of life. In: P. Gilbert, & J. Miles (Eds), *Body Shame: Conceptualisation, Research and Treatment*. New York: Brunner-Routledge.

Moos, R., & Schaefer, J. (1984). The crisis of physical illness: an overview and conceptual approach. In: R. Moos (Ed.), *Coping with Physical Illness: New Perspectives*, New York: Plenum, pp. 3–25.

Ng, C.H., & Schweitzer, I. (2003). The association between depression and isotretinoin use in acne. *Australian and New Zealand Journal Of Psychiatry*, **37**, 78–84.

Papadopoulos, L., Bor, R., & Legg, C. (1999a). Psychological factors in cutaneous disease: an overview of research. *Psychology, Health and Medicine*, **4**, 107–126.

Papadopoulos, L., Bor, R., & Legg, C. (1999b). Coping with the disfiguring effects of vitiligo: a preliminary investigation into the effects of cognitive-behavioural therapy. *British Journal of Medical Psychology*, **72**, 385–396.

Partridge, J. (1996). *Facial Disfigurement. The Full Picture.* London: Changing Faces.

Picardi, A., Abeni, D., Renzi, C., Braga, M., Puddu, P., & Pasquini, P. (2001). Increased psychiatric morbidity in female outpatients with skin lesions on visible parts of the body. *Acta Dermato-Venereologica*, **81**, 410–414.

Picardi, A., Abeni, D., Renzi, C., Braga, M., Melchi, C.F., & Pasquini, P. (2003a). Treatment outcome and incidence of psychiatric disorders in dermatological outpatients. *Journal of the European Academy of Dermatology and Venereology*, **17**, 155–159.

Picardi, A., Pasquini, P., Cattaruzza, M.S., Gaetano, P., Melchi, C.F., Baliva, G., Camaioni, D., Tiago, A., Abeni, D., & Biondi, M. (2003b). Stressful life events, social support, attachment security and alexithymia in vitiligo. *Psychotherapy and Psychosomatics*, **73**, 150–158.

Picardi, A., Pasquini, P., Cattaruzza, M.S., Gaetano, P., Baliva, G., Melchi, C.F., Tiago, A., Camaioni, D., Abeni, D., & Biondi, M. (2003c). Only limited support for a role of psychosomatic factors in psoriasis: results from a case-control study. *Journal of Psychosomatic Research*, **55**, 189–196.

Picardi, A., Pasquini, P., Cattaruzza, M.S., Gaetano, P., Baliva, G., Melchi, C.F., Papi, M., Camaioni, D., Tiago, A., Gobello, T., & Biondi, M. (2003d). Psychosomatic factors in first onset alopecia areata. *Psychosomatics*, **44**, 374–380.

Porter, J.R., & Beuf, A.H. (1988). Response of older people to impaired appearance: the effect of age on disturbance by vitiligo. *Journal of Aging Studies*, **2**, 167–181.

Porter, J.R., Beuf, A.H., Lerner, A., & Nordlund, J. (1986). Psychosocial effects of vitiligo. A comparison with 'normal' control subjects with psoriasis patients, and with patients with other pigmentary disorders. *Journal of the American Academy of Dermatology*, **15**, 220–224.

Rapp, S.R., Cottrell, C.A., & Leary, M.R. (2001). Social coping strategies associated with quality of life decrements among psoriasis patients. *British Journal of Dermatology*, **145**, 610–616.

Richardson, J. (1997). Chapter 10. In: R. Lansdown, N. Rumsey, E. Bradbury, T. Carr, & J. Partridge (Eds), *Visibly Different: Coping with Disfigurement*. Oxford: Butterworth-Heinemann.

Robinson, E., Rumsey, N., & Partridge, J. (1996). An evaluation of the impact of social interaction skills training for facially disfigured people. *British Journal of Plastic Surgery*, **49**, 281–289.

Root, S., Kent, G., & Al-Abadie, M.S.K. (1994). The relationship between disease severity, disability and psychological distress in patients undergoing PUVA treatment for psoriasis. *Dermatology*, **189**, 234–237.

Rumsey, N., Bull, R., & Gahagan, D. (1982). The effect of facial disfigurement on the proxemic behaviour of the general public. *Journal of Applied Social Psychology*, **12**, 137–150.

Rumsey, N., & Harcourt, D. (2004). Body image and disfigurement: issues and interventions. *Body Image*, **1**, 83–97.

Salzer, B., & Schallreuter, K. (1995). Investigation of personality structure in patients with vitiligo and a possible association with catecholamine metabolism. *Dermatology*, **190**, 109–115.

Samerotte, G.C., & Harris, M.B. (1976). The effects of actual and attempted theft, need, and a previous favor on altruism. *Journal of Social Psychology*, **99**, 193–202.

Shaw, W. (1981). Folklore surrounding facial deformity and the origins of facial prejudice. *British Journal of Plastic Surgery*, **34**, 237–246.

Scharloo, M., Kaptein, A.A., Weinman, J., Bergman, W., Vermeer, B.J., & Rooijmans, H.G.M. (2000). Patients' illness perceptions as predictors of functional status in psoriasis: a 1-year follow-up. *British Journal of Dermatology*, **142**, 899–907.

Tangey, J., & Fischer, K. (1995). *Self-Conscious Emotions. The Psychology of Shame, Guilt, Embarrassment and Pride.* New York: Guildford Press.

Thompson, A. (1998). *Exploring the Process of Adjustment to Disfigurement with Particular Reference to Vitiligo*. Unpublished doctoral thesis. University of Sheffield, UK.

Thompson, A., & Kent, G. (2001). Adjusting to disfigurement: processes involved in dealing with being visibly different. *Clinical Psychology Review*, **21**, 663–682.

Thompson, A.R., Kent, G., & Smith J.A. (2002). Living with vitiligo: dealing with difference. *British Journal of Health Psychology*, **7**, 213–225.

Van der Donk, J., Hunfield, J., Passcher, J., Knegt-Junk, K., & Nieber, C. (1994). Quality of life and maladjustment associated with hair loss in women with alopecia androgenetica. *Social Science and Medicine*, **38**, 159–163.

Wahl, A.K., Gjengedal, E., & Hanestad, B.R. (2002). The bodily suffering of living with severe psoriasis: in depth interviews with 22 hospitalised patients with psoriasis. *Qualitative Health Research*, **12**, 250–261.

Walters, E. (1997). Problems faced by children and families living with visible differences. In: R. Lansdown, N. Rumsey, E. Bradbury, T. Carr, & J. Partridge (Eds), *Visibly Different: Coping with Disfigurement*. Oxford: Butterworth-Heinemann.

Zhu, Y.I., & Stiller, M.J. (2001). Dapsone and sulfones in dermatology: overview and update. *Journal of the American Academy of Dermatology*, **45**, 420–434.

6

Skin disease and relationships

Litsa Anthis

'I remember a few months back, when I used to see his knuckles, how they were dry, cracked and bloody, and then I noticed his arm, and when I gently inquired … he would retreat and change the subject. This was also before we became close. He has slowly grown more comfortable and one night, after cuddling and holding each other for a while, he asked me if I'd like to see and I said please. He took off his shirt and I saw the extent of his condition. His entire back, arms and parts of his legs were red, with patches of dry skin and blood. It struck my heart, and I suddenly felt very close to him. I wasn't shocked or afraid, and I think he sensed that because he seemed to relax a little. I reached up and touched his shoulders and lightly stroked his back. He later told me he was grateful for how accepting I was, and how he hadn't been touched in a long time. His condition does not bother me, in fact, I admire him. He has a tremendous amount of strength. We have since been intimate, and while I do my best to make him feel comfortable, I can't seem to avoid situations that cause him pain; like when he rests his head on my chest when we lay together, and then he gets up, seeing the trail he has left on my black sweater … and I see the pain flash across his face. I don't know what to do. I reach up and kiss him, brush myself off, to show him it just goes away and say, "Black is not my best colour and yet I insist on wearing it!" He always smiles, but I can see how he carries his shame with him for the rest of the evening. *Partner of a patient with psoriasis.*'

In sickness and in health

When selecting a romantic partner, a personal choice is made based on reasons for wanting to be with a particular person. Some of these reasons are conscious and others are not. Undeniably, individual expectations and 'ideals' on what relationships should offer will vary, but for most there is a hope that existing or new relationships will serve as a source of support and personal growth (Altschuler, 1997). In the course of being together however, couples will face various difficulties that, if not negotiated and resolved, may threaten the quality of their relationship. The onset of skin disease can challenge the emotional, physical and social boundaries of a couple's existence. Sometimes like an uninvited guest it enters the relationship, and demands that it is incorporated into the couple's life (Rolland, 1994). Physical discomfort, disfigurement, embarrassment and social stigma (Gupta et al., 1993; Finlay & Coles,

1995; Kapp-Simon & McGuire, 1997; Kent, 2000) are but a few imposed realities. The implications on a couple will depend on how difficulties are contended with and resolved by both parties. Ideally, partners should support each other through sickness and in health; but if over time, disease-related stress expands opportunities for conflict and limits repertoires of support, relationship satisfaction is likely to decay.

Studies on couples and illness demonstrate that partner support is essential in the psychological adjustment to medical conditions such as cancer, cardiovascular disease and chronic pain (Pistrang et al., 1997). Support encouragement, requesting and accepting help, can facilitate adaptation and exert a positive influence over relationships (Rodin, 1982; Vaux, 1988; Heller & Rook, 1997). Such findings suggest that individual models of adjustment do not adequately account for the relational nature of coping observed in couples. In varying degrees, people do not only wish to enhance their own well-being but also that of their relationships with significant others (Coyne et al., 1990). According to Lyons et al. (1995a), understanding the relational nature of adjustment requires gaining insight into how a couple functions, communicates, integrates with others, and participates in work and leisure activities as indications of quality of life. Chronic illness can influence how a couple interacts by reducing the psychological or physical resources available in a relationship. This can lead to discomfort in communication, lessen support processes, and limit the range of activities couples share intimately and socially (Meyerowits et al., 1997). Burman and Mangolin (1992) have verified the value of focusing on specific couple variables, including couple interaction, relationship status, (whether one is in a significant relationship) and relationship quality (satisfied versus dissatisfied), in understanding health status.

In dermatology, the influence of intimate relationships on coping and adjustment is a neglected area of exploration, despite evidence that partners are an important source of support when facing ill health (Cutrona, 1996). Even less attention is paid to the partners of patients, who often do not know 'how to help', or are confused over what is 'the right thing to say or do', when a loved one is distressed over their skin. This chapter will explore the impact skin disease has on romantic relationships. Discussion will include coping with altered appearance, difficulties in communication, modified social networks and problems with sexual intimacy all of which, are potential triggers for acute and chronic stress in the life of a couple. Drawing from attachment theory, it will be proposed that attachment styles influence adjustment and how couples cope with the emotional distress that skin disease engenders.

Coping and adjustment

At the start of a potential relationship or in the course of an existing one, focusing on 'how we look' and 'want to appear' in the eyes of the other, can powerfully contribute to the chemistry of romance. Consequently, most individuals strive to manipulate their appearance in some way, so as to present themselves in the best possible light to prospective or current partners (Rumsey & Harcourt, 2004). The inability to enhance appearance due to skin disease creates an emotional reality that impacts on individual functioning, and can alter the matrix of social interaction (Koblenzer, 1987; Bradbury, 1996; Landsdown, 1997). Feelings of shame and increased self-consciousness may challenge an individual's sense of self, alter how they approach new romantic encounters or jeopardise emotional security in existing relationships. Research on coping and adjustment has identified clusters of difficulties that individuals commonly face, but there is no neat list of problems encountered by all patients (James, 1989). While skin disease can severely disrupt the lives of some individuals (Jowett & Ryan, 1985; Porter et al., 1990), the extent of disability and distress varies, and many patients report minimal suffering (Love et al., 1987; Blackney et al., 1988; Hunter et al., 1989; Landsdown, 1997.). Findings thus far have concluded the following; firstly, that disfiguring conditions have significant effects on depression, anxiety and self-esteem; secondly, there is a weak relationship between the severity of a condition and it's social and personal effects and thirdly, while treatment can reduce distress and improve quality of life, social improvements in patients lives are not closely related to clinical improvement (Kent, 2000).

Skin disease however, is not only an individual's problem. It is an interpersonal issue that has psychological consequences for both partners. Most couples share responsibility in solving difficulties (Skerrett, 1998), thus when one partner has a skin disease, it is important to know what kind of support is helpful? An interesting study of breast cancer patients and their partners revealed that following diagnosis, husbands provided greater support as their wives' physical impairment increased, but less support as wives' emotional distress increased (Bolger et al., 1996). This confirms the tendency among wives to engage in interpersonal and emotion-focused coping and a propensity among husbands to prefer interpersonal distance during periods of stress (Gottlieb & Wagner, 1991). Similar gender effects could operate in couples with skin disease, which suggests that emotional reactions to disfigurement, may at times, reduce chances of receiving empathic support when it is needed most.

When skin disease leads to relationship strain, it is not uncommon for patients to feel guilty for demanding more resources from their partner or to harbour fears of being rejected. Taking on the role of caregiver or care-receiver and no longer that of lover or partner can quickly destroy a couple's relationship (Gottlieb & Wagner, 1991; Schmaling & Sher, 1997). Psychological distress may also affect appraisal of the relationship itself. Sufferers who are in an upset mood often shift perspective towards the negative, and this can extend to perceptions of their partners. Research shows that when one partner is depressed, couples display more interpersonal negativity, report less relationship satisfaction and experience more stressful life events (Whiffen & Gotlib, 1989). Coping with the complexities of skin disease can thus test the commitment two people have towards one another by challenging both partners to work within new parameters. To consider couple relationships as merely providing beneficial support is overly simplistic (Schmaling & Sher, 2000). Couples also maintain loving relationships in order to meet the need for companionship and attachment.

Attachment styles

Originally attachment theory explained emotional bonds between infants and caregivers. Bowlby (1969–1980) believed attachment was a vital part of the human experience 'from the cradle to the grave' and that it played a powerful role in the emotional lives of adults. Hazan and Shaver (1987), developed Bowlby's theory further and noted that the major attachment styles described in the infant literature by Ainsworth et al. (1978); namely secure, avoidant and anxious- ambivalent were similar to how adults related in intimate relationships. Moreover, comparable behaviours became activated when adults were physically or perceived themselves to be psychologically separated from their partner. Romantic love can thus be conceptualized as an attachment process, but unlike infant attachment, it includes reciprocal behavioural systems of caregiving and sex (Shaver & Hazan, 1988).

Many relationship variables such as trust, communication and support correlate with secure and insecure patterns of relating. Avoidant adults, for example, need distance in a relationship and thus limit closeness to preserve autonomy; a need for self-sufficiency also means that they do not easily accept support from a partner. Anxious-ambivalent adults, desire intimate relationships but find them stressful and are often reluctant to raise or expose their needs and vulnerabilities to partners. Generally, adults with insecure styles of attachment communicate more negative and less positive emotions to partners (Simpson, 1990) and their attributions on partner behaviour during and after relationship conflict tends to exacerbate their anxiety (Simpson et al., 1996). In comparison, secure individuals are more trusting in relationships and higher in self-confidence than their insecure peers (Feeney & Noller, 1990). They are more comfortable with intimacy, being dependent on others, and worry less about abandonment (Collins & Read, 1990). They are also more likely to seek physical and emotional support from partners when distressed (Crowell et al., 1999) and provide support to upset partners. Adults characterized by a secure attachment style thus desire intimate relationships and seek to create within them a balance of closeness and autonomy (Simpson et al., 1992; Campbell, 2003).

Main et al. (1985) have likened attachment styles to 'working models' that shape cognitive, emotional and behavioural responses to others. These working models operate largely outside awareness, are relatively stable, resistant to change and centre on the regulation and fulfilment of attachment needs. The attachment framework is thus useful in differentiating attachment styles that typify healthy and troubled relationships (Collins & Read, 1994). When one partner faces illness however, it does not mean that previous difficulties and relationship struggles simply disappear. In this sense the attachment framework is beneficial in that it elucidates why some individuals with skin disease can use an intimate relationship as a secure-base to address disease-related difficulties such as feelings of shame over appearance or sexual problems and why other individuals struggle to communicate, or choose not to convey, their level of distress.

Appearance, attraction and shame

Romantic couples spend exclusive time together, they share social and leisure experiences, and allow themselves to be mutually vulnerable in ways they rarely do with others. Consequently, the feelings and perceptions romantic partners have about one another and the feedback they give on each other's appearance could substantially impact on how each will feel about themselves, their bodies and their relationship (Tantleff-Dunn & Gokee, 2002). Sixteen per cent of dermatology patients investigated by Hughes et al. (1983) reported that their skin condition affected their married life; Lannigan and Coterill (1989) found that a small proportion of women (9%) would not reveal their birthmarks, even to their husbands, and according to Koo (1996), many patients with psoriasis claim that their disease is a major obstacle in forming and sustaining intimate relationships. This demonstrates that, in both established and new relationships, disfigurement can be profoundly shaming if skin disease creates insecurities over how attractive and desirable individuals feel they are to their partners.

Kellet (2002) describes patients' responses to disfigurement as reflecting a specific form of body shame, namely dermatological shame, where focus is on the appearance of the skin and its relative attractiveness. Dermatological shame may be 'specific' to the disease or 'generalised' in relation to self-schemas (beliefs about the self). In specific dermatological shame, the focus is on the disease itself. Other aspects of the self remain unaffected and the individual is able to function effectively in various spheres of life. Individuals with a secure attachment style, being confident with their identity, are more likely to experience 'specific' shame. This would involve accepting the disease and dealing with its physical and psychosocial consequences in a contained way.

Generalised shame, as it suggests, is more pervasive. It merges with other shame schemas to create an all-encompassing inner experience of self-disgust that includes negative self-beliefs, social stigma and unfavourable comparisons with others. Such shame can have devastating effects on a couple if it leads to loss of intimacy and communication difficulties. For example, anxious-ambivalent adults naturally worry about abandonment, thus generalized shame may confirm that they are unattractive and ultimately rejectable. Fear of losing the relationship may then trigger coping, such as heightened displays of distress possibly to elicit a response from their partner or solicitous behaviour to gain acceptance. Avoidant adults are more likely to react by hiding their shame and by minimising displays of emotional distress over appearance.

In some couples, unaffected partners can deepen psychological distress in their loved one by passing insensitive comments about their appearance. Off-the-cuff remarks such as 'what happened to your face?' or those said in the heat-of-the-moment, such as 'your skin looks awful', can lead to relationship tension. Anxious-ambivalent individuals are particularly sensitive to criticism, thus a situation of high reactivity may evoke counter-attacking arguments in which partners begin to use each other's imperfections as weapons for war. Such conflict increases the likelihood of misunderstandings and, if it escalates, relationship distress will undermine the emotional security of both partners. Conversely, partners' who show unconditional acceptance, demonstrate respect, sensitivity, use humour and make their loved one feel valued and attractive, despite the skin condition, can have a powerful effect on adjustment. Richards et al. (2004) examined illness representations in patients with chronic psoriasis and their partners. Findings showed that divergent beliefs over the emotional impact of the disease was linked with significantly higher levels of anxiety, depression and worry in patients as opposed to their partners. 'Empathic coping' is thus a special challenge to partners as it involves understanding how dermatological shame impacts on their loved one and also on the functioning of the relationship.

Difficulties in communication

Secrecy and self-disclosure are two opposite forms of communication that can alter couple functioning by shaping what issues couples' feel able to discuss with one another and how needs for closeness and separateness are managed (Feeney & Noller, 1996). Secrecy in skin disease involves safety behaviours such as making excuses to avoid activities involving exposure of the skin and concealing affected areas through the use of clothes or cosmetics. In existing relationships, even if a skin condition is openly acknowledged, secrecy may operate if conversations about the disease are subtly avoided. Partners may be equally anxious over what to say or how to set a fitting tone of conversation without saying the wrong thing and potentially embarrassing themselves or their partner. Sometimes, the location of a condition is not immediately apparent, thus the decision as to whether or when to tell a new romantic partner can be delayed (Papadopoulos & Walker, 2003). Ginsburg (1996) argues that the status of a patient's self-esteem and body image prior to disease onset is clinically important in determining how they are likely to cope with an altered appearance. Secrecy may lessen opportunities for embarrassment (Miles, 2002) however, as a communication strategy, it reflects significant anxiety related to appearance (Kent & Thompson, 2002). Cosmetic products are useful for many patients in that they lower anxiety by improving appearance, which in turn can increase self-confidence regarding romantic acceptance (Leary & Kowalski, 1995). There is a danger however that if improved self-esteem stimulates further interest in appearance, 'camouflaging' may become a psychological tool for maintaining social functioning (Meli & Giorgini, 1984).

Avoidant Attachment Style: 'I never leave the house without makeup, even if it's to go to the shop next door. On a bad day, I won't even leave my bedroom without makeup (I live with three men). What I hate is the time it takes. People always make fun of me (in a nice way …) about how long it takes me to get ready and I wish I could be ready in 5 minutes because applying all the makeup is really a problem. Sometimes it takes up to half an hour. I know I can look great with make-up on, and no one even notices I have a problem if I'm covering it up, but I live in terror of people seeing how I "really" look. I won't go swimming in the summer and when I'm dating someone (as I am now) I make up a million excuses as to why they can't stay the night, to the point of ruining the relationship. I don't want to have to tell everyone in my life … how insecure I am about the way I look' (Female acne patient).

In contrast, self disclosure is a communication strategy that aims to curtail the fear of 'being seen', or 'being discovered'. Mikulincer and Nachshon (1991) investigated the relationship between attachment style and self-disclosure in couples. They found that secure and anxious-ambivalent individuals reported more self-disclosure than avoidant individuals, and secure adults showed the most reciprocity and flexibility over the range of issues discussed with partners.

Secure Attachment Style: 'As far as relationships go, my personal opinion is that my partner would have to be comfortable with my skin because it plays such a huge part in my life. Also, being honest and open about things at the beginning of a relationship avoids any embarrassing and "nasty" surprises further on down the line. I don't expect non-eczema suffers to understand completely the emotions I experience, but I would like them to be a bit compassionate about my condition, especially if I'm going to have a long-term relationship with them' (Female eczema patient).

Self-disclosure is a central provision in intimate relationships (Monsour, 1992), however, certain individuals prefer not to threaten their relationship with self-presentations of depression and anxiety, even if that is their emotional state. 'Being open' carries the risk of being judged as poorly adjusted (Glick et al., 1974) and this is especially so when society tends to admire people who 'bear their cross' (Lyons et al., 1995a). For some individuals or couples, hiding emotional distress or avoiding conflict acts as a form of 'protective buffering' that may minimize disruption in a couple's relationship and lifestyle. This style of coping depicts how couples use different strategies to try to protect their relationship during times of stress (Coyne & Smith, 1991).

Changes in social networks

In the course of their relationship, couples create substantial social contexts that involve sharing domestic, recreational or occupational activities. When skin disease changes companionship in any one of these areas, the maintenance or nature of the relationship may be threatened (Lyons & Sullivan, 1998). Changes in a couple's social network may occur through reduced interactions with others and an increase in companionate activities at home (Morgan et al., 1984). More than often, withdrawal is a response to the damaging effects of social stigma. Porter et al. (1990) reported that vitiligo patients experienced embarrassment and anxiety when meeting strangers and that many had been victims of rude remarks in the face of public ignorance. In the short term, avoidance may serve a protective function, but it may also lead to loss of friendships and activities that would typically increase a couple's social network. In an early survey, Jobling (1976) asked 186 members of the British Psoriasis Association what they considered was the worst aspect about having psoriasis? Eighty-four per cent alluded to isolation based on their difficulties in establishing social contacts, and forming relationships. Negative changes in lifestyle will stress a relationship further, if a couple's ability to function as a unit is continually challenged.

For some couples, skin disease brings new responsibilities into a relationship and this may be taxing if traditional gender roles become unbalanced (Danoff-Burg & Revenson, 2000). For example, in one affected couple, a wife had to seek employment when her husband was unable to continue his job at a dry cleaner because the steam and chemicals aggravated his eczema. Functional limitations may also lead to changes in a couple's leisure activities; for instance, patients with psoriasis receiving psoralen plus ultraviolet light (PUVA) treatment often sacrifice holidays in the sun. If, for the sake of the relationship, partners also forgo valued activities, they too are in danger of becoming isolated through their own loss of freedom. Firstly, by missing out on social interactions that were previously shared and secondly, by having to do more things alone. At times the more intimate the relationship, the increased likelihood of mutual isolation.

Relationship functioning is thus shaped by a couple's desire and competence in readjusting shared activities and social networks to increase companionship. Successful adaptation may involve downplaying the disease as a constraint, focusing on the present and not allowing disfigurement to assume a dominant place in the relationship. Positive readjustment may also include network remodelling, which involves finding and adding resources such as support groups, to existing networks (Lyons & Meade, 1995b). According to Locker (1983) such changes reflect 'legitimacy' in illness, namely having others accept the reality and nature of constraints that are placed on the affected couple.

Body image and sexual intimacy

Another important area in a couple's relationship is that of sexual intimacy. The association between body image and sexual functioning is a good illustration of the reciprocal nature of interpersonal influences in skin disease (Weiderman, 2002). Common sense dictates that good sex is about confidence, feeling good about yourself and your body. Yet, many dermatology patients struggle with physical intimacy and often have sex lives that are fraught with difficulties.

Avoidant Attachment Style: 'I'm a 23 year-old male and I have psoriasis on my chest, back, butt, arms and legs. Fortunately it is not on my hands, face, in my hair or on my privates. People don't know I have it because I keep all the evidence covered. I've been dating a girl for 6-months and we were getting serious but I still hadn't told her about my psoriasis. I didn't know how to do it. Then I read this forum and got some courage. I think she had been waiting for me to take the plunge about sex for a long time, so finally. … I suggested it and just said, "But there's something you have to know." She knew nothing about psoriasis and cooled right away. … I got as far as showing her one arm and that was the end of it. Now I feel so low, I don't know whether to dump her because she's so closed-minded or to just give up.'

A negative body image can damage the perception of self as a sexual being and thus disrupt intimacy in a relationship. Gupta and Gupta (1997) investigated the impact of psoriasis on the sexual activities of 120 sufferers and found that 40% experienced a decline in sexual activity and had higher scores on depression than non-affected patients. Embarrassment over unsightly or painful lesions was most apparent during intercourse; which also confirms past research that sexual functioning is disrupted in dermatology patients if genital areas are affected (Buckwalter, 1982; Medansky, 1986). It appears that negative body image perpetuates sexual difficulties because anxiety or low self-esteem can decrease a patients' interest in initiating or being receptive to sexual activity (Weiderman, 2002). Furthermore, feelings of shame and depression are often exacerbated if affected individuals interpret sexual difficulties as reflecting their undesirability to their partner (Tantleff-Dunn & Gokee, 2002).

In 2003, a US marketing firm surveyed 502 patients with psoriasis on their attitudes towards relationships; 38% reported difficulties with sex and intimacy. It was evident that problems were more prevalent in young single adults as 53% reported difficulties in their sex life, in contrast to 30% of married subjects. Furthermore, 49% of adults aged 18–24 and 36% of adults aged 25–35 experienced angst in intimate situations. Dermatological shame was also prevalent since 52% turned off the lights when intimate with their partner and 48% worried that their partner was embarrassed by their psoriasis. On the issue of relationship functioning, 26% said psoriasis interfered with their ability in getting emotionally close with their partner. Interestingly, a different study of vitiligo patients and their beliefs on intimate relationships revealed that most patients felt more embarrassed in non-sexual interpersonal relationships than in intimate sexual relationships (Porter et al., 1990). Both these studies and the excerpt provided at the start of this chapter (from the partner of a patient with psoriasis), illustrate that couple relationships can have a protective effect but that good communication is critical to ensuring sexual confidence.

Relationship-focused coping

In exploring the impact that skin disease has on couples, it appears that successful coping not only depends on the ability to problem-solve difficulties or regulate emotions, but also on the regulation and adjustment of relationships. Efforts directed at maintaining a relationship or to attending to the emotional needs of a partner have been referred to as relationship-focused coping (Lyons et al., 1995a). Empathy, for example, is a central dimension of adult attachments (Story & Bradbury, 2004); in couples where one partner has skin disease, relationship-focused coping may entail re-evaluating and changing perspective on what is important in the relationship, such as placing less emphasis on appearance (Lyons et al., 1995a). Coping efforts will undoubtedly vary from couple to couple, but adjustment can include behaviours such as support-giving and support-receiving, legitimacy and communal coping to help both partners cope over time.

Skin diseases that are punctuated by periods of exacerbation and remission can stress individual and relationship functioning. When the skin 'flares', even if it is only visible to the patient, feelings of imperfection (Ginsburg, 1996) can turn normal couple activities, such as having sexual relations or undressing in each other's company into sources of stress. Attachment styles are also triggered by acute or chronic stress, thus it is under these conditions that differences in attachment behaviour are likely to be more pronounced (Simpson et al., 1992). If the disease spreads, or worsens, secure individuals are able to seek the support or reassurance they need from partners. 'Active engagement' in such couples entails coping jointly with difficulties by discussing feelings or engaging in interpersonal problem-solving (Coyne & Smith, 1991). In contrast, avoidant adults are more likely to become distant or withdrawn. Simpson et al. (1992) argue that in reality, avoidant individuals *want* to be physically and emotionally close to their partners but are afraid of this intimacy. It is theorised that at lower levels of distress (maybe during remission), avoidant individuals can display behaviours and emotions that achieve greater intimacy and relationship satisfaction. However, as levels of anxiety increase they become fearful and cannot tolerate closeness. This explains, perhaps, why avoidant individuals are unwilling to turn to their partners for support or even provide support when needed. The nature of support-seeking and support-giving behaviours in relationships may thus also be influenced by the degree of anxiety that skin disease engenders.

Various aspects of coping can also be shared with other significant relationships in a couple's network. Communal coping refers to the process whereby close friends or family members make skin disease 'our problem' and thus cope with the emotional and instrumental aspects of the disease with the patient. Consequently, in times of stress, friends and family are expected to help. From the patient's perspective, adopting a communal orientation involves developing greater concern for the welfare of others; this may include considering how disfigurement, for example, influences the coping of family or friends in social situations. This change in focus, often leads to less self-involvement (Lyons et al., 1995a), promotes communication, and can enhance mutual problem-solving. It is also a form of legitimacy as it involves having others accept the reality and nature of constraints that are placed on the couple (Locker, 1983). What constitutes legitimacy in a relationship however is a complex issue. In some couples, self-disclosure which is aimed at increasing intimacy, may fail to secure legitimacy, particularly if the unaffected partner deems the expressed distress as 'over the top' in relation to the severity of the skin condition. In other couples, legitimacy is reinforced when a partner 'empathically' withdraws in periods of high stress to allow the sufferer to deal with their upset rather than engage in conversations that could escalate distress. Legitimacy will undeniably be influenced by the nature of a couple's attachment styles; but for some patients the strongest legitimacy comes from external relationships that are fostered with co-sufferers or from dermatology web sites that provide anonymous forums for discussing physical, psychological and relationship problems. Bradbury (1996) states that support groups can be very helpful in legitimising distress, so long as they do not create a niche of people who reinforce their sense of difference.

Conclusion

This chapter has explored the impact skin disease has on couples and how attachment styles can influence the process of adjustment. It is evident that altered appearance, difficulties in communication, shifts in social networks and decreased sexual intimacy are triggers for acute and chronic stress that can threaten relationship functioning. Despite the aforementioned difficulties, the process of adjustment also provides couples with opportunities to discover untapped potential in their relationship and to deepen their commitment and intimacy (Story & Bradbury, 2004). The advantage of using an attachment-based theoretical perspective in skin disease is that, whilst explaining normative relational processes, it considers the variation of adults' experiences in romantic relationships and highlights how couples become and remain distressed in the course of coping with the demands and consequences of various skin diseases.

The attachment perspective also incorporates tenets of social and personality psychology, which are having an increasing influence in psychodermatological research; firstly, by acknowledging that a set of mechanisms (working models) contribute to individual stability and secondly, by highlighting that social and environmental factors can powerfully influence attachment behaviour (Feeney & Noller, 1996). The notion of relationship-focused coping (De Longis & O'Brien, 1990) expands understanding of dyadic influences in skin disease by stressing that successful adjustment is not solely dependent on the ability to problem-solve or regulate emotions, but also on the regulation of intimate relationships. An interesting point to consider is that since attachment patterns are relatively stable in 70% of individuals, (Baldwin & Fehr, 1995; Fuller & Fincham, 1995) it can be conjected that the 30% who change their attachment style may be doing so as a result of a romantic relationship. By extension, individuals who potentially might have been devastated by skin disease may be coping successfully because of their partner. Currently, investigators are calling for greater attention to relational factors in coping with chronic illnesses, however a comprehensive model that addresses the stresses, strategies and outcomes of relationship-focused coping is still evolving (Feeney & Noller, 1996). Lawrence et al. (1998) have proposed that attachment styles can change through couple therapy. For example, couples prone to escalating negative exchanges in times of stress could benefit from improved conflict resolution. Couples in which one partner is prone to depression may benefit from learning how to provide greater emotional support. Further research on relationship-focused coping could thus explore what processes protect couples from the stresses of skin disease and examine how the interplay of dyadic coping and individual adjustment changes over the course of a relationship. Maintaining this focus of investigation is fundamental in that, medical care that neglects how individual's feel in the 'real world' (Goleman, 1995) and in the 'reality' of their most intimate relationships, is no longer adequate for the 'comprehensive' treatment of skin disease.

REFERENCES

Ainsworth, M.D.S., Blehar, M.C., Waters, E. & Wall, S. (1978). *Patterns of Attachment: A Study of the Strange Situation*. Hillsdale, NJ: Lawrence Erlbaum.

Altschuler, J. (1997). Gender and illness: implications for family therapy. *Journal of Family Therapy*, **15**, 381–401.

Baldwin, M.W. & Fehr, B. (1995). On the instability of attachment style ratings. *Personal Relationships*, **2**, 247–261.

Bolger, N., Foster, M., Vinokur, A.D., & Ng, R. (1996). Close relationships and adjustment to a life crisis: the case of breast cancer. *Journal of Personality and Social Psychology*, **70**, 283–294.

Bowlby, J. (1969–1980). Attachment and loss. London: Hogarth Press, pp. 129.

Blackney, P., Herndon, D., Desai, M., Beard, S., & Wales-Seale, P. (1988). Long-term psychological adjustment of children after severe burn injury. *Journal of Burn Care and Rehabilitation*, **11**, 472–475.

Bradbury, E. (1996). *Counselling People with Disfigurement*. Leicester: BPS Books.

Buckwalter, K. (1982). The influence of skin disorders on sexual expression. *Sex Disability*, **5**, 98–106.

Burman, B., & Mangolin, G. (1992). Analysis of the association between marital relationship and health problems: an interactional perspective. *Psychological Bulletin*, **112**, 39–63.

Campbell, D.B. (2003). The relationships among negative self-schemas, partner attachment styles, and relationship adjustment. *Dissertation Abstracts International: Section B: The Science and Engineering*, **64(2B)**, 1001.

Collins, N.L., & Read, S.J. (1990). Adult attachment, working models, and relationship quality in dating couples. *Journal of Personality and Social Psychology*, **58**, 644–663.

Collins, N.L., & Read, S.J. (1994). Cognitive representations of attachment: the structure and function of working models. In: K. Bartholomew, & D. Perlman (Eds), *Advances in personal relationships*. London: Jessica Kingsley, pp. 53–90.

Coyne, J.C., & Smith, D.A.F. (1991). Couples coping with myocardial infarction: I. a contextual perspective on wives' distress. *Journal of Personality and Social Psychology*, **6**, 404–412.

Coyne, J.C., Ellard, J.H., & Smith, D.A. (1990). Social support, interdependence, and the dilemmas of helping. In: B.R. Sarason, I.G. Sarason, & G.R. Pierce (Eds), *Social Support: An Interactional View*. New York: John Wiley, pp. 129–149.

Crowell, J., Fraley, R.C., & Shaver, P.R. (1999). Measures of individual differences in adolescent and adult attachment. In: J. Cassidy, & P.R. Shaver (Eds), *Handbook of Attachment: Theory, Research, and Clinical Applications*. New York: Guilford Press, pp. 434–465.

Cutrona, C.E. (1996). Social support as a determinant of marital quality: The interplay of negative and supportive behaviors. In: G.R. Pierce, B.R. Sarason, & I.G. Sarason (Eds), *Handbook of Social Support and the Family*. New York: Plenum, pp. 173–194.

Danoff-Burg, S., & Revenson, T.A. (2000). In: K.B. Schmaling, & T.G Sher (Eds), *The Psychology of Couples and Illness*. Washington: American Psychological Association, pp. 105–133.

De Longis, A., & O'Brien, T. (1990). An interpersonal framework for stress and coping: an application to the families of alzheimers patients. In: M.A.P. Stephens, S.E. Hobfoll, D.L. Tennebaum, & J.H. Crowther (Eds), *Stress and Coping in Later Life Families*. Washington: Hemisphere, pp. 221–239.

Feeney, J.A., & Noller, P. (1990). Attachment style as a predictor of adult romantic relationships. *Journal of Personality and Social Psychology*, **58**, 281–291.

Feeney, J.A., & Noller, P. (1996). *Adult Attachment*. London: Sage.

Finlay, A.Y., & Coles, E.C. (1995). The effect of severe psoriasis on the quality of life of 369 patients. *British Journal of Dermatology*, **132**, 236–244.

Fuller, T.L., & Fincham, F.D. (1995). Attachment style in married couples: relation to current marital functioning, stability over time, and method of assessment. *Personal Relationships*, **2**, 17–34.

Ginsburg, I.H. (1996). The psychosocial impact of skin disease: an overview. *Psychodermatology*, **14(3)**, 473–484.

Glick, I.O., Weiss, R.S., & Parkes, C.M. (1974). *The First Years of Bereavement*. New York: John Wiley.

Goleman, D. (1995). *Emotional Intelligence*. London: Bloomsbury.

Gottlieb, B.H., & Wagner, F. (1991). Stress and support processes in close relationships. In: J. Eckenrode (Ed.), *The Social Context of Coping*. New York: Plenum, pp. 165–188.

Gupta, M.A., & Gupta, A.K. (1997). Psoriasis and sex: a study of moderately to severely affected patients. *International Journal of Dermatology*, **36**, 359–362.

Gupta, M., Schork, N., & Gupta, A. (1993). Suicidal ideation in psoriasis. *International Journal of Dermatology*, **32**, 188–190.

Hazan, C., & Shaver, P.R. (1987). Romantic love conceptualised as an attachment process. *Journal of Personality and Social Psychology*, **52**, 511–524.

Heller, K., & Rook, K.S. (1997). Distinguishing the theoretive functions of social ties. In: S. Duck (Ed.), *Handbook of Personal Relationships*, 2nd edn. Chichester, England: Wiley, pp. 648–670.

Hughes, J., Barraclough, B., Hamblin, L., & White, J. (1983). Psychiatric symptoms in dermatology patients. *British Journal of Psychiatry*, **143**, 51–54.

Hunter, J.A.A., Savin, J.A., & Dahl, M.V. (1989). *Clinical Dermatology*. London: Blackwell Scientific Publishing.

James, P. (1989). Dermatology. In: A.K. Broome (Ed.), *Health Psychology*. London: Chapman and Hall, pp. 183–207.

Jobling, R.G. (1976). Psoriasis: a preliminary questionnaire study of sufferer's subjective experience. *Clinical Experimental Dermatology*, **1**, 233–236.

Jowett, S., & Ryan, T. (1985). Skin disease and handicap: An analysis of the impact of skin conditions. *Social Science and Medicine*, **20(4)**, 425–429.

Kapp-Simon, K., & McGuire, D. (1997). Observed social interaction patterns in adolescents with and without craniofacial conditions. *Cleft Palate-Craniofacial Journal*, **34**, 380–384.

Kellet, S. (2002). Shame-focused acne: a biopsychosocial conceptualisation and treatment rationale. In: P. Gilbert, & J. Miles (Eds), *Body Shame: Conceptualisation, Research and Treatment*. East Sussex: Brunner-Routledge, pp. 135–154.

Kent, G. (2000). Understanding the experiences of people with disfigurements: an integration of four models of social and psychological functioning. *Psychology, Health and Medicine*, **5(2)**, 117–129.

Kent, G., & Thompson, A. (2002). The development and maintenance of shame in disfigurement: implications for treatment. In: P. Gilbert, & J. Miles (Eds), *Body Shame*. Hove: Brunner-Routledge, pp. 103–116.

Koblenzer, C.S. (1987). *Psychocutaneous Disease*. Orlando: Grune & Stratton.

Koo, J. (1996). Population based epidemiologic study of psoriasis with emphasis on quality of life assessment. *Psychodermatology*, **14(3)**, 485–496.

Landsdown, R.L., Rumsey, N., Bradbury, E., Carr, T., & Partridge, J. (1997). *Visibly Different: Coping with Disfigurement*. Oxford: Butterworth-Heinemann.

Lannigan, S., & Coterill, J. (1989). Psychological disabilities amongst patients with port wine stains. *British Journal of Dermatology*, **121**, 209–215.

Lawrence, E., Eldridge, K.A., & Christensen, A. (1998). The enhancement of traditional behavioural couples therapy: consideration of individual factors and dyadic development. *Clinical Psychology Review*, **18(6)**, 745–764.

Leary, M., & Kowalski, R. (1995). *Social Anxiety*. London: Guildford Press.

Locker, D. (1983). *Disability and Disadvantage: The Consequences of Chronic Illness*. London: Tavistock.

Love, B., Byrne, C., Roberts, J., Browne, G., & Brown, B. (1987). Adult psychosocial adjustment following childhood injury: the effect of disfigurement. *Journal of Burn Care and Rehabilitation*, **8**, 280–285.

Lyons, R.F., & Meade, D. (1995b). Painting a new face on relationships: relationship remodelling in response to chronic illness. In: S. Duck, & J.T. Wood (Eds), *Confronting Relationship Challenges*. London: Sage, pp. 181–210.

Lyons, R., & Sullivan, M. (1998). Curbing loss in illness and disability: a relationship perspective. In: J.H. Harvey (Ed.), *Perspectives on Personal and Interpersonal Loss: A Sourcebook*. Bristol: Taylor & Francis, pp. 137–152.

Lyons, R.F., Sullivan, M.J.L., Ritvo, P.G., & Coyne, J.C. (1995a). *Relationships in Chronic Illness and Disability*. Thousand Oaks, California: Sage.

Main, M., Kaplan, N., & Cassidy, J. (1985). Security in infancy, childhood and adulthood: a move to the level of representation. *Monographs of the Society for Research in Child Development*, **50(1–2)**, 66–104.

Medansky, R. (1986). Psoriasis and sexuality. *Medical Aspects of Human Sexuality*, **20**, 144–149.

Meli, C., & Giorgini, S. (1984). Aesthetics in psychosomatic dermatology: 1. Cosmetics, self image and attractiveness. *Clinics in Dermatology*, **2(4)**, 180–187.

Meyerowits, B.E., Levin, K., & Harvey, J.H. (1997). On the nature of cancer patient's social interactions. *Journal of Personal and Interpersonal Loss*, **2**, 49–69.

Mikulincer, M., & Nachshon, O. (1991). Attachment styles and patterns of self-disclosure. *Journal of Personality and Social Psychology*, **61**, 321–331.

Miles, J. (2002). Psoriasis: the role of shame on quality of life. In: P. Gilbert, & J. Miles (Eds), *Body Shame: Conceptualisation, Research and Treatment*. Hove: Brunner- Routledge, pp. 119–134.

Monsour, M. (1992). Meanings of intimacy in cross and same-sex friendships. *Journal of Social and Personal Relationships*, **9**, 277–295.

Morgan, M., Patrick, D.L., & Charlton, J.R. (1984). Social networks and psychosocial support among disabled people. *Social Science and Medicine*, **19**, 489–497.

Papadopoulos, L., & Walker, C. (2003). *Understanding Skin Problems.* London: John Wiley & Sons.

Pistrang, N., Barker, C., & Rutter, C. (1997). Social support as conversation: analysing breast cancer patient's interactions with their partners. *Social Science and Medicine*, **45(5)**, 773–782.

Porter, J.R., Beuf, A.H., Lerner, A., & Nordlund, J. (1990). The effect of vitiligo on sexual relationships. *Journal of the American Academy of Dermatology*, **22**, 221–222.

Richards, H.L., Fortune, D.G., Chong, S.L.P., Manson, D.L., Sweeney, S.K.T., Main, C.J., & Griffiths, C.E.M. (2004). Divergent beliefs about psoriasis are associated with increased psychological distress. *Journal of Investigative Dermatology*, **123(1)**, 49–56.

Rodin, M.J. (1982). Non-engagement, failure to engage, and disengagement. In: S. Duck (Ed.), *Personal Relationships.* London: Academic Press, pp. 31–49.

Rolland, J.S. (1994). Families, *Illness and Disability: An Integrative Treatment Model.* New York: Basic Books.

Rumsey, N., & Harcourt, D. (2004). Body image and disfigurement. *Body Image*, **1**, 83–97.

Schmaling, K.B., & Sher, T.G. (1997). Physical health and relationships. In: W.K. Halford, & H.J. Markman (Eds), *Clinical Handbook of Marriage and Couples.* New York: Wiley, pp. 323–345.

Schmaling, K.B., & Sher, T.G. (2000). *The Psychology of Couples and Illness.* Washington: American Psychological Association.

Shaver, P.R., & Hazan, C. (1988). A biased overview of the study of love. *Journal of Personality and Social Psychology*, **5**, 473–501.

Simpson, J.A. (1990). Influence of attachment styles on romantic relationships. *Journal of Personality and Social Psychology*, **59**, 971–980.

Simpson, J.A., Rholes, W.S., & Nelligan, J.S. (1992). Support seeking and support giving within couples in an anxiety-provoking situation: The role of attachment styles. *Journal of Personality and Social Psychology*, **62**, 434–446.

Simpson, J.A., Rholes, W.S., & Alonso, D. (1996). The impact of conflict on close relationships: An attachment perspective. *Journal of Personality and Social Psychology*, **71**, 899–914.

Skerrett, K. (1998). Couples adjustment to the experience of breast cancer. *Family, Systems and Health*, **16(3)**, 281–298.

Story, L.B., & Bradbury, T.N. (2004). Understanding marriage and stress: Essential questions and challenges. *Clinical Psychology Review*, **23**, 1139–1162.

Tantleff-Dunn, S., & Gokee, J.L. (2002). Interpersonal influences on body image development. In: T.F. Cash, & T. Pruzinsky (Eds), *Body Image: A Handbook of Theory, Research and Clinical Practice.* London: Guildford Press, pp. 108–124.

Vaux, A. (1988). *Social Support: Theory, Research, and Intervention.* New York: Praeger.

Weiderman, M.W. (2002). *Body image* and sexual functioning. In: T.F. Cash, & T. Pruzinsky (Eds), *Body Image: A Handbook of Theory, Research and Clinical Practice.* London: Guildford Press, pp. 108–124.

Whiffen, V.E., & Gotlib, I.H. (1989). Stress and coping in maritally distressed and non-distressed couples. *Journal of Social and Personal Relationships*, **6**, 327–344.

Acknowledgements

The author acknowledges the Internet reference for US study: www.looksmart.com PR Newswire 09/02/04 (Title: Survey shows impact of psoriasis is more than skin deep; self-confidence, relationships, work/school and social interactions affected) and the quotes from patients taken from forums on skin disease on the Internet.

7

The impact of skin disease on children and their families

Penny Titman

Skin disease is very common among children and young people. For example, up to 20% of young children develop eczema and the majority of young people develop some symptoms of acne temporarily during adolescence (McHenry et al., 1995; Smithard et al., 2001). However, there is surprisingly little research on the psychological impact of skin disease in childhood and the focus of most research in paediatric psychology has been on life-threatening conditions, such as cancer. Despite the lack of research, there is widespread acknowledgement of the impact of skin disease on the psychological well-being and quality of life of children, and increasing awareness of the importance of understanding the psychological impact of skin disorders on children and their families (Howlett, 1999).

This chapter will start by outlining some key issues in understanding the relationship between skin disorders and psychological factors for children. This includes the importance of considering both a developmental and systemic framework for childhood problems, and potential difficulties that may arise in communicating with a child about sensitive topics, such as how they feel about their appearance. The chapter will then describe current theoretical models of the psychological impact of physical disease on children and their families, and how these inform our understanding of the impact of skin disease. The next section will review research on the impact of skin conditions on the relationship between a mother and her baby or child, and the impact of skin conditions on the child's self-esteem. Finally, intervention strategies and methods of improving the psychological outcome for children and their families will be reviewed.

In order to understand the impact of skin disease on children it is essential to consider both the child's developmental stage and the context in which they live. The impact of a skin condition will vary considerably depending on the age and level of independence of the child. Young children are entirely dependent on their parents for their healthcare and a young child's response to a skin condition is therefore likely to both be influenced by, and have a strong influence on, the response of their parents. However, as the child grows up, they will be more strongly influenced by their peer group and become less dependent on their parents. As a consequence of this, the implications for a child with, for example, severe eczema at the age of 2 years are very different from the implications for an adolescent of age 14. Whilst for the 2-year-old child, their relationship with their parent and the parent's skills in managing the condition may be very important factors, for the adolescent, the important issues are more likely to be related to their self-esteem, their sense of belonging to their peer group and their own ability to care for their skin.

In most families, the child's mother acts as the main carer for the child and this seems to be particularly true for families where a child has a physical illness (Sloper, 2000). Research has therefore focused on the relationship between the child and his or her mother. For this reason, mothers are referred to as the main carers throughout this chapter. However, it is likely that the many of the same findings may also apply to fathers if they were in the main caring role in a family.

The developmental stage of the child will also affect the best way to communicate with the child about concerns regarding their skin. Very young children are unlikely to be able to put their concerns into words and it is often necessary to rely on parental report or to use pictures or drawings as a way of communicating. However, as the child gets older and becomes more independent, they will often prefer to talk about concerns without their parent present. In particular, adolescents may appear non-communicative if seen with their parents, but will often talk much more freely about their concerns if seen on their own. It is important for anyone working with children with skin conditions to be flexible about how they see the child and his or her family in order to ensure they are able to communicate as effectively as possible with the child. Nonetheless, the sensitive nature of the child's concerns may make it very hard for them to discuss these in a brief consultation with someone they do not know well and they may be reluctant to report concerns spontaneously.

The impact of skin disease on the psychological well-being of the child and family

There are a large number of studies that have shown that any form of physical illness during childhood increases the risk of psychological difficulties for the child (Lavigne & Faier-Routman, 1992; Wallander & Varni, 1998). There is also evidence from a few studies about the specific impact of a skin disorder on childhood psychological problems. For example, Absolon et al. (1997) found that children with eczema had higher rates of behavioural problems than healthy children. Rates of psychological difficulties are even higher among young people with acne and up to a half of 12–20-year olds with acne have been shown to have psychological or social problems (Smithard et al., 2001).

Early studies in this field focused on measuring levels of psychological distress, or the presence or absence of psychological difficulties in the child or parent. However, whilst the presence or absence of psychological distress or disorder is one important outcome measure, it is quite a narrow way of defining psychological adjustment. Hence there has been increased interest in other types of outcome measure, such as quality of life, to attempt to encompass other important areas of experience, such as social and educational factors.

There are now several measures of quality of life for skin conditions that have been developed specifically for children and which help us to access the child's view of the impact of a skin condition on themselves. For example, the Children's Dermatology Life Quality Index (Lewis-Jones & Finlay, 1995) is a generic assessment tool for use with all skin conditions and it comes in both a cartoon and a written version (Holme et al., 2003). It consists of 10 questions about the impact of the child's skin condition on their everyday life, such as taking part in leisure activities or going to school. This measure has proved very useful in providing a way of comparing the impact of different types of skin conditions on children from the child's own viewpoint. For example, atopic eczema has consistently been shown to have a high impact on quality of life of children (Chuh, 2003). The highest scores reported using this measure have been for the very rare form of dystrophic epidermolysis bullosa (Horn & Tidman, 2002). Other disease-specific measures of quality of life have been used as part of treatment evaluation (Fehnel et al., 2002).

These measures of quality of life have proved useful because it becomes possible to assess the impact of a skin condition from the child's own viewpoint. It is also then possible to compare across different conditions, or to compare the impact of different types of the same condition, as well as to evaluate the impact of treatment from the child's viewpoint.

Theoretical models of the psychological impact of skin disease during childhood

Most theoretical models of child and family adaptation to chronic illness use a stress and coping model adapted from Lazarus and Folkman (1984) to explain the impact of a chronic illness on children and their families. For example, Wallander and Varni's (1998) model predicts that disease-related variables (such as severity or visibility), functional independence and psychosocial stressors can be seen as risk factors, whereas intrapersonal factors (such as coping style), social–ecological factors and stress processing are all seen as resistance factors.

However, most of the research studies to date have been cross-sectional, descriptive studies. Unfortunately, these research designs may not capture the complexity of the processes that may be involved, particularly when trying to understand relationships between people and causal processes. For example, the reciprocal relationship between a mother and her child, particularly when it involves both the mother and child's psychological and physical state, is a very complex one and has sometimes been oversimplified. It is not possible to disentangle the direction of causality in a cross-sectional study and this means that a degree of caution is required when interpreting many studies. A biopsychosocial model, such as the one described by Howlett (1999), which takes into account the influences that biological, social and psychological factors have on both the child and his or her carer, and the possibility of reciprocal causal patterns is the most useful way of trying to understand the interrelationship of these factors.

However, the exact nature of the risk factors that are important predictors of which children adjust well to their condition and which children do develop psychological difficulties are not well understood. Whilst intuitively, severity of the condition would seem to be a good predictor, this is not always supported by research. The very concept of severity is quite a complex one – some conditions are considered 'severe' because they are life threatening, such as cancer, whilst others may not be life threatening but do have a big impact on 'quality of life' and are therefore severe in a different way. Skin conditions are rarely severe in the sense of 'life threatening' in children. However, they often have a very big impact on the child's quality of life and that of his or her family, and may be seen as 'severe' in terms of the impact on day-to-day life. It has become clear that there is no simple relationship between the severity of a condition as assessed 'objectively' by a clinician and psychological adjustment.

The visibility of the child's condition is also thought to have an impact on the child's adjustment to their condition. Many skin conditions are immediately apparent to other people and children, and their families have to manage the reaction of other people to the child's condition on a daily basis. Papadopoulos et al. (2000) compared the impact of acne which was mainly on a young person's body with acne mostly on the face, and showed that the visible, facial acne sufferers had lower self-esteem and that their body image was more affected than if it was on their body.

The impact of skin disease on the mother–child relationship

For a very young child or baby who is dependent on his or her mother for all his or her care, there is likely to be a reciprocal relationship between the mother and child in terms of both the child's physical and psychological state. For example, if a baby is distressed or fretful because of physical discomfort, this may result in an increased need for care from his or her mother, and this increased demand on the mother's caring resources may make her feel more stressed and she may respond less positively towards her baby. The complex interrelationships between the mother's physical and psychological state, and the babies' physical and psychological state need to be recognised although it has been hard to separate out these different influences in research.

There are several ways in which the mother–child relationship may be affected by a child with a skin condition. For conditions that are present at birth but were not necessarily expected (e.g. birthmarks or epidermolysis bullosa), the physical appearance of the child's skin can be very distressing. The mother's immediate reaction may well be of shock and she is likely to need some time and possibly support to adjust to this. There is considerable variation between mothers on how they respond to a skin condition, depending on factors related to the appearance of the baby, and the mother's own beliefs and attitudes towards physical appearance (Walters, 1997). Whilst for some mothers, a skin condition can undoubtedly make it harder for her to bond with her child, for mothers who bond well it can lead to an increased feeling of protectiveness towards the child arising out of the need to protect a more 'vulnerable' child. In the long term it is important for the mother to be able to find an appropriate balance between caring for her child and allowing the child to develop his or her own resources for dealing with difficult situations arising from a skin condition.

In addition, physical contact between a mother and her baby are very important for the developing relationship. If the baby or child has a skin condition which is painful or uncomfortable this may have an impact on the quality of physical contact between the mother and child (Koblenzer, 1990). In some cases, if the treatment requires a lot of skin contact, for example, applying moisturisers or other topical medication, or if the child requires a lot of physical contact to soothe them and reduce their discomfort, this can result in additional physical contact between mother and child, although the quality of this contact may still be affected if the child is uncomfortable and finds the treatment procedures unpleasant. Bick (1986), described the psychoanalytic treatment of a child with eczema and emphasised the importance of the mother's ability to 'contain' the child's discomfort and drew a parallel between this and the mother's role in managing a young infant's behaviour.

There are few empirical studies which assess the relationship between a mother and child with a skin condition but Solomon and Gagnon (1987) carried out an observational study which compared the relationship between mothers and healthy children with mothers of children with eczema. They found that mothers of children with eczema touched, soothed and stroked their babies as much as mothers of healthy children and that, contrary to their expectations, the babies were not more distressed or difficult to soothe than the babies in the control group. However, they did find that the mothers and babies with eczema had fewer episodes of positive interactions, which would be worth examining in a future study.

Gil et al. (1988) also carried out an observational study and showed an important relationship between scratching behaviour and parental response to scratching. In particular, this study indicated that scratching actually increased during periods when parents asked the children not to scratch, and decreased during times when the child was actively involved in tasks or when parents attended to other appropriate behaviour by the child.

It has often been assumed in the past that difficulties accepting a child with a skin condition may result in a disruption to the attachment of the child to his or her parent. Attachment is the normal process through which a young child forms a close relationship with their caregiver and which is thought to provide the basis for the development of subsequent relationships (Bowlby, 1980). This initial relationship provides the child with a secure base and enables the child to explore the world safely and confidently, and therefore increase independence. If the child feels upset or threatened, this important relationship acts as a secure base to which the child can return and be comforted. In order for the child to develop a secure attachment to the primary caregiver, the mother needs to be able to be sensitive to the child's needs and responsive to them.

There is also very little evidence from empirical studies about the effect on the child's attachment to his or her mother as a result of a skin condition. Daud et al. (1993) tested the hypothesis that young children with eczema are more insecurely attached to their mothers than healthy children using the strange situation procedure (Ainsworth et al., 1978). Contrary to expectation, they found no differences in the security of the child's attachment to his or her mother between the children with eczema and their control group of healthy children. However, these mothers did report difficulties in their relationship with their child in terms of parenting and reported finding it hard to discipline their child effectively and on parent report questionnaires they did identify higher rates of behavioural problems amongst their children compared to healthy children.

The balance of evidence suggests that the presence of a skin condition does not always result in difficulties in the mother–child relationship, but that for some mothers and children difficulties may develop. These mothers will need sympathetic understanding of their difficulties with their baby and it is important that any difficulties are not seen as the mother's 'fault' and she does not feel blamed for these difficulties. Too often the mother is seen as 'rejecting' her child or dismissed as unable to bond with her child, whereas she may need help and understanding to overcome her own fears and anxieties about her child's appearance. Developing the mother's confidence in handling her baby and managing any treatment is very important, as is enabling her to manage other people's reactions confidently. Encouraging direct physical contact can help; for example, by using simple massage techniques (Schachner et al., 1998). Mothers often find it very helpful to talk to others with the same condition, especially if the condition is very rare and is likely not to be well understood by most people (Clarke, 1999).

In addition, any physical treatment plan needs to be clearly demonstrated and time spent with the mother discussing her concerns. Nurse-led clinics have been shown to be very effective in terms of improving the mother's understanding of the child's condition and her use of prescribed treatment (Cork et al., 2003) and this in turn can lead to improved management of the condition and reduced severity of the condition. Several studies have indicated high levels of dissatisfaction about the conventional medical treatment offered to children with skin problems, and this leads to low levels of adherence to prescribed treatments and expensive use of alternative or complementary treatments (Ernst, 2000). Skin care routines are complex and can be time consuming, and it is essential to ensure that enough guidance is given at the time treatment is prescribed if it is to be used effectively.

There is good evidence that caring for a child with a skin condition, such as eczema, places additional demands on mothers and that the common problems of young children (such as sleeping, eating and behaviour problems) can be more difficult to manage with a young child with eczema (Elliott & Luker, 1997; Pauli-Pott et al., 1999). The additional demands of the physical skin care routine can result in high levels of parental stress and have a marked impact on the quality of life for the family (Lawson et al., 1998; Warschburger et al., 2004). Parents of young children with eczema report that they find parenting their child more difficult as a result of the eczema and may need additional help with strategies for managing sleep difficulties or common behavioural problems (Titman, 2003).

It is very important for the child that his or her mother is able to overcome high levels of anxiety and is able to manage the child's skin condition confidently. It is also important for the mother to feel she is able to love and fully accept her child despite any appearance difficulty. If the child's mother is able to become resolved about the child's condition, she is more likely to enable her child to develop a positive attitude towards his or her own skin, and develop a good sense of self-esteem. She will also be in the best position to deal with any anxieties or difficulties her child has in a constructive way.

The impact of skin conditions on self-esteem

It is hard for a child to grow up with a skin condition and for this not to have some impact on their self-esteem. However, the variation in the impact on self-esteem cannot be entirely attributed to the severity of the child's condition, because it is very dependent on psychological factors and the child's beliefs about their condition. It is possible for a child with very damaged skin to report high levels of self-esteem and vice versa; for a young person with very trivial skin blemishes to report a considerable impact on self-esteem.

Self-esteem has been most studied in relation to acne and studies have clearly demonstrated that adolescents with acne do have lower self-esteem than non-affected adolescents (Papadopoulos et al., 2000; Smith, 2001). Unfortunately, one of the more effective types of medication used for acne has been linked with concerns about depression and suicide in young people, although the evidence as to the drug's causal role in this is not clear as yet. Given the high rate of depression and suicidal ideation amongst adolescents in general, and adolescents with acne in particular, the treatment with isotretinoin needs to be carefully monitored to ensure fluctuations in mood are identified and if necessary can be modified (Hull & D'Arcy, 2003).

Young children are not usually self-conscious about their appearance, but self-consciousness tends to increase as the child grows up and most adolescents are acutely self-conscious. As a child gets older they have to leave the safe confines of the family home and manage the transition first to nursery or playgroup, then to primary school and then to secondary school. These transitions can be extremely difficult for a child with a skin condition who has to cope with other people's reaction to their skin including considerable amounts of curiosity and intrusive comments. Most young people or adults who have grown up with a skin condition can recall extremely unpleasant and traumatic episodes of being teased or excluded as a consequence of their skin condition (Richardson, 1997).

Unlike adults, young children will often stare openly at a child who looks different, and will sometimes make hurtful comments or ask questions in quite a disinhibited way. In addition, they will often react with disgust or horror without any attempt to disguise their reaction because it may upset the person concerned. Young children have been shown to have clear preferences for children who look attractive and so a child who is visibly different can easily feel rejected or excluded by his or her peers (Sigelman et al., 1986). Managing these types of reactions can be very difficult for a young child with a skin condition and may result in them becoming increasingly self-conscious. This will obviously have an impact on the child's self-esteem but can also set up a 'negative mind set' which results in the child becoming increasingly sensitive to other's comments and at worst withdrawing from or avoiding social situations because of this.

It is important for teachers and parents to help dispel some of the fears that other children or parents may have about the child's skin condition. Common misperceptions are that the condition may be contagious or may be very painful if the skin looks red or inflamed. Before the child starts at school it is important for the parent to meet with the child's teacher to explain the condition and to provide information about it, particularly if it is very rare or if the condition may be affected by factors within the school, such as temperature or sitting on a carpet. If appropriate, the teacher can spend some time with the whole class helping them to understand the condition and promoting friendships.

All schools should have anti-bullying policies in place and should have plans to help reduce bullying in school. However, there is considerable variation in how well these are implemented and how proactive schools are in promoting and managing differences within the school. There are some excellent training packages available for teachers from organisations, such as Kidscape, as well as Changing Faces and the National Eczema Society.

Nonetheless, the child will face some incidents of teasing and may well find it helpful to develop strategies for managing these incidents. There has been very little research specifically on evaluating such interventions for children with skin disorders. However, Bradbury (1996), and Kish and Lansdown (2000) have evaluated programmes for children with disfigurements of various origins. These concentrate on developing social skills to help children manage social situations more confidently, as it is often the case that children may approach a situation without much confidence and be more likely to expect a negative reaction. They also help children to develop self-protection strategies, such as imagining a force field around themselves which can deflect negative comments. Whilst these programmes have not been evaluated formally, they do appear to help improve the child's sense of mastery over teasing incidents and improve their self-esteem.

Older children, particularly young adolescents, can also use some of the stress management techniques and cognitive–behavioural therapy techniques used for adults (Stangier & Ehlers, 2000). Some of the habit reversal techniques that have been found to be useful for adults can be applied to children, but they do need some adaptation to make them useful and may not be so successful since they rely on high levels of motivation (Bridgett et al., 1996).

Accessing psychological services for children with skin conditions

It can be very difficult to access appropriate services for children with skin conditions who have psychological difficulties (Czyzewski & Lopez, 1998). Very few paediatric dermatology services will have a liaison service with a psychologist or other mental health professional. There is considerable resistance among many families to the prospect of a referral to a psychology or mental health service, partly because of the stigma attached to mental health difficulties but also because many parents will feel they are being blamed for not managing the child's condition well enough or that they are not good enough as parents. It is also often the case that local community-based child mental health services are not able to accept referrals of children who have these type of adjustment difficulties, because they have to give priority to more pressing mental health difficulties. Although many parents do experience caring for a child with a physical condition as stressful, they will usually feel the stress is caused by the skin condition itself and therefore think that psychological approaches are not likely to be of benefit.

This can be a very difficult topic to discuss directly with a family and requires sensitive handling. It is important to take a non-judgemental approach and to explain how the psychology service may be relevant to the child's condition. It can help to acknowledge the fears the family may have about such a referral. Given the sensitive nature of many of the adolescent or young people's concerns, it may be necessary to talk this through with the young person on their own, to try and improve the chances of them taking up the referral. It helps to be very clear with the family about the way in which the psychology service would expect to work with them, and to give a clear reason for the referral making it very clear that this is not a judgement on them as parents and is intended to be helpful to them.

Dermatitis artefacta (skin damage caused deliberately) is occasionally seen in children, and is a complex condition that requires careful management to engage the child and family. Rogers et al. (2001) describe a series of 32 young people seen with artefactual skin conditions and emphasise the importance of good liaison between the mental health worker and the dermatologist. It can be very difficult to get the family to accept the referral and it is important to avoid confrontation as this can result in the family withdrawing the child.

Summary

There are still relatively few studies of the psychological impact of skin disease on children and families, and very little formal evaluation of therapeutic input. However, the awareness of the impact of skin conditions on the quality of life of both the child and his or her family has led to increased acknowledgment of the importance of addressing these difficulties. This in turn should lead to improved services for children and families, which integrate psychological approaches with medical treatment strategies.

REFERENCES

Absolon, C.M., Cottrell, D., Eldridge, S.M., & Glover M.T. (1997). Psychological disturbance in atopic eczema: the extent of the problem in school aged children. *British Journal of Dermatology*, **137**, 241–245.

Ainsworth, M.D.S., Blehar, M.C., Waters, E., & Wall, S. (1978). *Patterns of Attachment*. Hillsdale, NJ: Erlbaum.

Bick, E. (1986). Further considerations on the function of the skin in early object relations: findings from infant observations integrated into child and adult analysis. *British Journal of Psychotherapy*, **2**, 292–299.

Bowlby, J. (1980). *Attachment and Loss: Vol. III Loss*. New York: Basic Books.

Bradbury, E. (1996). *Counselling People with Disfigurement*. Leicester: British Psychological Society.

Bridgett, C., Noren, P., & Staughton, R. (1996). *Atopic Skin Disease: A manual for Practitioners*. Basingstoke: Wrightson Biomedical Publishing.

Chuh, A.A.T. (2003). Quality of life in children with pityriasis rosea: a prospective case control study. *Pediatric Dermatology*, **20**, 474–478.

Clarke, A. (1999). Psychosocial aspects of facial disfigurement: problems, management and the role of a lay-led organisation. *Psychology, Health and Medicine*, **4**, 127–142.

Cork, M.J., Britton, J., Butler, L., Young, S., Murphy, R., & Keohane, S.G. (2003). Comparison of parent knowledge, therapy utilisation and severity of atopic eczema before and after explanation and demonstration of topical therapies by a specialist dermatology nurse. *British Journal of Dermatology*, **149**, 582–589.

Czyzewski, D.I., & Lopez, M. (1998). Clinical psychology in the management of pediatric skin disease. *Dermatologic Clinics*, **16**, 619–629.

Daud, L.R., Garralda, M.E., & David, T.J. (1993). Psychosocial adjustment in preschool children with atopic eczema. *Archives of Disease in Childhood*, **69**, 670–676.

Elliott, B.E., & Luker, K. (1997). The experiences of mothers caring for a child with severe atopic eczema. *Journal of Clinical Nursing*, **6**, 241–247.

Ernst, E. (2000). The usage of complementary therapies by dermatological patients: a systematic review. *British Journal of Dermatology*, **142**, 857–861.

Fehnel, S.E., McLeod, L.D., Brandman, J., Arbit, D.I., McLaughlin-Miley, C.J., Coombs, J.H., Martin, A.R., & Girman, C.J. (2002). Responsiveness of the acne specific quality of life questionnaire (Acne-QoL) to treatment for acne vulgaris in placebo-controlled clinical trials. *Quality of Life Research*, **11**, 809–816.

Gil, K.M., Keefe, F.J., & Sampson, H.A. (1988). Direct observation of scratching behavior in children with atopic dermatitis. *Behavior Therapy*, **19**, 213–227.

Holme, S.A., Man, I., Sharpe, J.L., Dykes, P.J., Lewis-Jones, M.S., & Finlay, A.Y. (2003). The children's dermatology life quality index: validation of the cartoon version, *British Journal of Dermatology*, **148**, 285–290.

Horn, H.M., & Tidman, M.J. (2002). Quality of life in epidermolysis bullosa. *Clinical and Experimental Dermatology*, **27**, 707–710.

Howlett, S. (1999). Emotional dysfunction, child–family relationships and childhood atopic dermatitis. *British Journal of Dermatology*, **140**, 381–384.

Hull, P.R., & D'Arcy, C. (2003). Isotretinoin use and subsequent depression and suicide: presenting the evidence. *American Journal of Clinical Dermatology*, **4**, 493–505.

Kish, V., & Lansdown, R. (2000). Meeting the psychosocial impact of facial disfigurement. *Clinical Child Psychology and Psychiatry*, **5**, 497–512.

Koblenzer, C.S. (1990). A neglected but crucial aspect of skin function: a challenge for the 90s. *International Journal of Dermatology*, **29**, 185–186.

Lavigne, J.V., & Faier-Routman, J. (1992). Psychological adjustment to pediatric physical disorders: a meta-analytic review. *Journal of Pediatric Psychology*, **17**, 133–157.

Lawson, V., Lewis-Jones, M.S., Finlay, A.Y., Reid, P., & Owens, R.G. (1998). The family impact of childhood atopic dermatitis: the dermatitis family impact questionnaire. *British Journal of Dermatology*, **138**, 107–113.

Lazarus, R.S., & Folkman, S. (1984). *Stress, Appraisal and Coping*. New York: Springer.

Lewis-Jones, M.S., & Finlay, A.Y. (1995). The children's dermatology life quality index (CDLQI): initial validation and practical use. *British Journal of Dermatology*, **132**, 942–949.

McHenry, P.M., Williams, H.C., & Bingham, E.A. (1995). Management of atopic eczema. *British Medical Journal*, **310**, 843–847.

Papadopoulos, L., Walker, C., Aitken, D., & Bor, R. (2000). The relationship between body location and psychological morbidity in individuals with acne vulgaris. *Psychology Health and Medicine*, **5**, 431–438.

Pauli-Pott, U., Dauri, A., & Beckmann, D. (1999). Infants with atopic dermatitis: maternal hopelessness, child-rearing attitudes and perceived infant temperament. *Psychotherapy and Psychosomatics*, **68**, 39–45.

Richardson, J. (1997). Chapter ten. In: R. Lansdown, N. Rumsey, E. Bradbury, T. Carr, & J. Partridge (Eds), *Visibly Different: Coping with Disfigurement*. Oxford: Butterworth-Heinmann.

Rogers, M., Fairely, M., & Santhanam, R. (2001). Artefactual skin disease in children and adolescents. *The Australasian Journal of Dermatology*, **42**, 264–270.

Solomon, C.R., & Gagnon, C. (1987). Mother and child characteristics and involvement in dyads in which very young children have eczema. *Developmental and Behavioural Paediatrics*, **8**, 213–220.

Schachner, L., Field, T., Hernandez, R.M., Duarte, A.M., & Krasnegor, J. (1998). Atopic dermatitis symptoms decreased in children following massage therapy. *Pediatric Dermatology*, **15**, 390–395.

Sigelman, C.K., Miller, T.E., & Whitworth, L.A. (1986). The early development of stigmatising reaction to physical differences. *Journal of Applied Developmental Psychology*, **7**, 17–32.

Sloper, P. (2000). Predictors of distress in parents of children with cancer: a prospective study. *Journal of Pediatric Psychology*, **25**, 79–91.

Smith, J.A. (2001). The impact of skin disease on the quality of life of adolescents. *Adolescent Medicine*, **12**, 343–353.

Smithard, A., Glazebrook, C., & Williams, H. (2001). Acne prevalence, knowledge about acne and psychological morbidity in mid adolescence: a community based study. *British Journal of Dermatology*, **145**, 274–279.

Stangier, U., & Ehlers, A. (2000). Stress and anxiety in dermatological disorders. In: D.I. Mostofsky, & D.H. Barlow (Eds), *The Management of Stress and Anxiety in Medical Disorders*. Needham Heights, MA: Allyn and Bacon, pp. 304–333.

Titman, P. (2003). *Understanding Childhood Eczema*. Chichester: John Wiley and Sons.

Wallander, J.L., & Varni, J.W. (1998). Effects of pediatric chronic physical disorders on child and family adjustment. *Journal of Child Psychology and Psychiatry*, **39**, 29–46.

Walters, E. (1997). Problems faced by children and families living with visible difference. In: R. Lansdown, N. Rumsey, E. Bradbury, T. Carr, & J. Partridge (Eds), *Visibly Different: Coping with Disfigurement*. Oxford: Butterworth-Heinmann.

Warschburger, P., Buchholz, H. Th., & Petermann, F. (2004). Psychological adjustment in parents of young children with atopic dermatitis: which factors predict parental quality of life? *British Journal of Dermatology*, **150**, 304–311.

8

Psychological therapies for dermatological problems

Linda Papadopoulos

Introduction

The enormous growth in the last two decades in cosmetic surgery, dieting and the fashion industry are all the indicators of the huge investment that society puts into the 'appearance industry'. In the western world, people are subjected to the same message constantly: 'Attractive people are popular, happy, successful, interesting and are often loved and worshipped' (Papadopoulos & Walker, 2003). Of course, cosmetic and physical perfection are rarely associated with those experiencing cutaneous conditions. Consequently, people with dermatological illnesses are left feeling minimised as individuals, tend to be highly sensitive to the social significance of their actions and appearance, to anticipate rejection by others, and to experience embarrassment and/or shame (Kellett & Gilbert, 2001).

Therefore, it is not surprising that due to their visibility and appearance-altering quality, skin disorders have important psychological implications for the sufferer, making the long-established link between psychological factors and dermatology even stronger. Yet, little attention has been paid to them or to the ways in which to address them. Indeed, as the prevalence and aetiology of the majority of skin diseases are neither well known nor understood by the general public, dermatological ailments are often surrounded by misconceptions and stigma.

The link between dermatological and psychological problems has long been prominent in the published literature. Dermatology has a distinct relation with psychosomatics as the skin has strong psychological implications. The skin is a complex system made up of glands, blood vessels, nerves and muscle elements, many of which are controlled by the autonomic nervous system and can be influenced by psychological stimuli. These have the capacity to cause autonomic arousal and are capable of affecting the skin and the development of various skin disorders. Several theories postulate psychophysiological mechanisms underlying various dermatological disorders (Papadopoulos & Bor, 1999). Indeed, not only do the skin and psyche share their embryonic origin but they are also closely inter-twined functionally (Van Moffaert, 1992). There also appears to be a relationship between the skin and the immune system. Clinical studies have shown that psy-chological stress can cause suppression of killer T-cells and macrophages, both of which play important roles in skin-related immune reactions (Papadopoulos et al., 1999). Another important link between the dermis and the psyche is that skin diseases may signal internal pathogenic processes.

On a more practical level, dermatology deals with an organ that can be readily seen and touched. This has consequences for how a patient interacts with their lesions and also for the lack of privacy that so many complain about. From intru-sive questions to rude comments, the visibility of cutaneous conditions has a devastating effect on the need for many to keep their condition private or personal. Consequently, a skin disease brings with it a variety of life changes and challenges for the patient, as our society places much emphasis on looks and appearance.

This chapter will aim to outline some of the core psychosocial issues faced by people living with skin diseases in the context of the use of counselling to address them and review the most frequently used psychological treatments. Their efficacy will be critically evaluated. Finally, recommendations for treatment will be made taking into account the potential challenges faced by people with skin problems.

Psychosocial impact of skin diseases

Within the psychodermatological literature, there is a great degree of consensus that skin disorders have a negative impact upon the psychological and emotional functioning of some patients. Indeed, research has provided evidence that such appearance-altering diseases can have profound behavioural, emotional and cog-nitive impact upon sufferers (Griffiths & Richards, 2001; Thompson & Kent, 2001). A brief overview of the most commonly researched psychological implications is thus provided.

Damaged skin often carries the connotation of contagion or a lack of hygiene (Van Moffaert, 1992). Owing to a lack of health education and awareness in derma-tology, some associate skin disease with such issues. This ignorance means that a skin disease patient may find that some people react negatively towards them or treat them differently because of the way they look. Consequently, the sufferer may experience distress, feel stigmatised and thus begin to avoid certain social activities that either involve the revealing of the lesions, such as swimming, or that involve potential intimacy with a third party, such as dating or physical displays of affection.

In their qualitative study with vitiligo patients, Thompson et al. (2002) found that the central recurring theme in their interviews concerned perceived differ-ences from previous appearance and from others. Common behavioural strategies used by these patients were concealment and avoidance, which were mostly utilised in order to avoid negative reactions from others. Moreover, acne patients have been shown to limit exposure through social avoidance and to conceal skin lesions (Kellett & Gilbert, 2001). Psoriasis patients have also been found to engage in anticipatory and avoidance coping behaviours, which are unrelated to the severity of their condition and this is hypothesised to relate to stigmatisation and rejection (Griffiths & Richards, 2001). Like previous work on disfigurement and social anxiety, skin disease patients use these dysfunctional behavioural strategies to manage the impression they make on others and their frequent use illustrates the overriding concerns about social exclusion (Thompson et al., 2002).

Cognitively appearance-altering, cutaneous conditions can have a profound effect on self-concept and on body image. Any minor deformity or disfigurement can contribute to the development of heightened body awareness. Cutaneous conditions can often have a progressive and episodic course making it necessary for the patient to adapt to changes in physical appearance. Hence, patients must not only learn to cope with the challenges of living with an appearance that deviates from the norm but also to adapt to a changing body image. That is, skin disease patients must develop and maintain a sense of self-esteem without relying upon physical attractiveness. This is an extremely difficult task given the fact that the robust relationship between self-esteem and body image has been underscored in numerous studies (Papadopoulos et al., 2002).

Feelings of anxiety, uncertainty and helplessness are often cited by dermatology patients as accompanying the diagnosis of their skin condition. Without the knowledge of when or how the condition will develop, the patient may be left wondering about what behaviours or actions might be contributing to its progression. Moreover, dermatology patients experience heightened self-consciousness, which, in turn, has negative implications for interpersonal interactions and relationships. Research has shown that self-consciousness is a common reaction amongst acne patients (Kellett & Gilbert, 2001). Papadopoulos et al. (1999b) found a significantly high frequency in irrational, negative thoughts among vitiligo patients.

Studies have also highlighted a higher prevalence of psychiatric disorder in dermatology patients (Hughes et al., 1983). Although it seems a little premature to make links between dermatological disorders and psychiatric conditions based solely on evidence from cross-sectional designs, research has certainly reported the increased prevalence of conditions, such as anxiety and depression in this population. Gupta et al. (1993) found that over 5% of their sample of psoriasis patients had active suicidal ideation and almost double this figure had expressed the wish to die. Similarly, Fortune et al. (2000) found that psoriasis patients had worry scores on standardised assessment indicative of pathological worrying, with 25% of the entire sample scoring above the mean for patients with a definite diagnosis of generalised anxiety disorder. A linkage between obsessive–compulsive disorder (OCD) and dermatology has also recently been investigated. There is a specific clinical condition, *acne excoriee*, which is characterised by excessive picking and/or scratching of real or imagined lesions which is considered to be a dermatological variant of OCD (Kellett & Gilbert, 2001). Acne patients may also use too much soap or other vigorous cleaning methods in order to address the feelings of infection. Hence this type of behaviour may qualify as a compulsion.

As well as affecting psychosocial functioning, negative psychosocial experiences may also affect the onset and progression of cutaneous conditions. Clinical observations have suggested that stress often precedes the onset or exacerbation of many dermatological conditions that share both psychosomatic and immunological components, such as vitiligo, psoriasis and atopic dermatitis (Koblenzer, 1983; Al-Abadie et al., 1994). For example, emotional distress and stressful life events have been suggested as contributory factors in the onset of vitiligo (Papadopoulos et al., 1998).

Despite such overriding evidence concerning the impact of skin disease on the sufferer and its implicated role in aetiology, cutaneous conditions are not generally recognised as a handicap and people with such conditions often face trivialisation of their distress (Papadopoulos & Walker, 2003). Until recently, little attention was given to the psychological effects of skin conditions and the challenges faced by those who suffer from them, not only by family and/or friends but by health professionals. Since skin diseases are rarely life threatening, their impact is often minimised by health professionals. Some doctors tend to make judgements about the seriousness of a medical condition in terms of pathological severity rather than quality of life. They consequently deem many skin conditions trivial or unimportant. Patients are left feeling misunderstood or embarrassed for having taken up their doctor's time. They may also feel that they are not taken seriously or are upset by being trivialised. Hence, consultations with professionals can become quite problematic (Papadopoulos & Walker, 2003).

Of course, individual variation exists with regard to adjustment to skin disease and some people cope well with their condition. However, there exists a proportion of this population that finds it particularly difficult to cope (Papadopoulos & Bor, 1999). Clearly then, psychodermatological research has only recently begun to identify the factors that might account for successful adjustment to disfigurement. Variables, such as coping, social support and cognitive representations of illness are being investigated in order to account for psychological impact (Fortune et al., 2000; Papadopoulos et al., 2002; Thompson et al., 2002). Such research has obvious theoretical and therapeutic implications. Theoretically, any model designed to explain psychological adjustment to skin conditions will need to provide explanations for the relationship between disease and psychological distress. Therapeutically, an understanding of patients' adjustment to disease will firstly help professionals to understand patients' attitudes towards treatment and care, and improve the chances of benefiting from them. Secondly, it will elucidate patients' attitudes and representations of their illness as well as their seeking, and adherence to, treatment (Papadopoulos et al., 2002).

Psychological approaches to treatment for dermatological conditions

Increasingly then, within the dermatological literature, attention was given to the therapeutic benefits that might derive from psychological interventions beyond those of standard medical care. Given the close and clear associations between psychological factors and cutaneous conditions, it is not surprising that the effects of such treatment have been investigated. The literature has documented psychological interventions for a number of cutaneous conditions, such as vitiligo, psoriasis, acne and atopic dermatitis, which have been suggested to be as effective for each of these types of disorders as classical medical procedures (Van Moffaert, 1992; Papadopoulos & Bor, 1999). For example, in their review of psychological therapies for the treatment of psoriasis, Winchell and Watts (1998) describe a case in which two psychiatric patients with psoriasis were given a suggestion that imipramine would have beneficial effects on their skin condition. Following this suggestion one of the patients experienced complete remission while the other improved significantly.

The methodological rigour of trials in this field has improved over time. Specifically, early research must be viewed as tentative in view of certain methodological shortcomings. It often used single-case experimental designs with few attempts to evaluate the progress of patients after the termination of therapy or to compare results with those of other patients or matched controls (Papadopoulos & Bor, 1999). Studies were also based on small samples with no control groups. Outcome measures were unsophisticated and were usually given by a single observer. Furthermore, outcome was measured by changes to either psychological or dermatological health but rarely by both. Since the early 1980s, psychocutaneous research investigating the efficacy of psychological interventions has started to employ controlled trials with large samples and quantitative cross-sectional designs, and to examine outcome from both psychological and dermatological perspectives (Papadopoulos & Bor, 1999).

Psychological approaches, such as psychoanalysis and hypnosis (Gray & Lawlis, 1982) as well as behavioural (Wolpe, 1980) and cognitive–behavioural therapy (Papadopoulos et al., 1999b) have been used to treat people affected by skin disorders (see Table 8.1). Indeed, such interventions have been shown to produce clinically significant improvements in cutaneous conditions, such as atopic dermatitis

Table 8.1. Approaches to treatment of dermatological conditions

	Behaviour therapy	Cognitive–behaviour therapy	Group therapy	Psychodynamic psychotherapy
Time frame	Here-and-now	Here-and-now	Here-and-now	Understanding the past, focuses on current relationships
Cost	Cost-effective	Cost-effective	Cost-effective	Expensive
Techniques	Systematic desensitisation, modelling, relaxation, habit-reversal training, assertiveness and social skills training, imagery	Problem-solving, cognitive restructuring, guided imagery, modelling	Psychoeducation, social and assertiveness skills training, role-play	Analysis of transference and counter-transference, hypnosis
Time	Short-term	Short-term	Short-term	Long-term
Efficacy	Psoriasis, eczema, vitiligo, acne	Psoriasis, eczema, vitiligo, acne	Psoriasis, eczema, vitiligo	Eczema

(eczema), psoriasis, vitiligo and virus-mediated diseases (Van Moffaert, 1992) and have helped patients to improve their psychological well-being and quality of life (Cole et al., 1988; Papadopoulos et al., 1999a). Outlined below are the main therapeutic techniques used in dermatology settings.

Behaviour therapy

Behaviour therapy incorporates applications derived from learning theory (classical and operant conditioning) and employs them to the treatment of persistent, maladaptive, learned habits. Among behaviour therapy techniques are systematic desensitisation, assertiveness and social skills training, behaviour analysis, relaxation training (e.g. autogenic and progressive muscle relaxation, biofeedback) habit-reversal training and imagery. The aim of these techniques is to progressively diminish maladaptive behavioural responses by repeatedly inhibiting the anxiety by means of competing responses (Wolpe, 1980). A behaviour analysis is conducted where the clinician collects information about the relationship between stimuli and behavioural responses in order to understand the role of anxiety.

Diverse behavioural therapeutic strategies have been applied, either separately or in combination with other psychological techniques to dermatological conditions.

Systematic desensitisation is an appropriate technique for the treatment of dermatoses which feature anticipatory anxiety (Van Moffaert, 1992). The fear and apprehension that patients with skin disease may feel about themselves may be challenged by this technique. Through graded exposure, the patient enters situations that they may fear and avoid. The *habit-reversal technique* is a common strategy used to inhibit scratching and it has been reported to have some success with skin disorders, such as eczema and psoriasis (Ginsburg, 1995). It involves self-monitoring for early signs and situational cues of scratching and practising alternative responses, such as clenching the fists (Ehlers et al., 1995). *Relaxation* has beneficial effects on skin disorders because it reduces stress levels. It is a useful way to help patients prepare for anxiety-provoking situations or to cope with stressful social predicaments. Relaxation can be used on its own as a means to reduce anxiety or tension or can be paired with imagery. There are various different techniques, such as progressive muscle relaxation or autogenic relaxation training.

Imagery with skin disease patients is employed in order to help them cope with anxiety relating to their condition. Imagery is a useful technique for helping the patient to visualise the feared situation while in a relaxed state (Papadopoulos & Bor, 1999). *Assertiveness and social skills training* is appropriate for patients with cutaneous conditions that attract attention from others, such as staring or personal questions. Interventions focus on improving social skills and ways of expressing emotions, thus helping patients deal more effectively with the reactions of others and learn a more positive mode of social functioning (Robinson et al., 1996).

Weinstein (1984) found that compared with patients receiving only medical treatment (psorasen plus ultraviolet light A, PUVA), both psychological treatment groups, one receiving progressive relaxation and guided imagery and the other meeting to discuss psychosocial concerns about psoriasis, were effective in reducing the signs and symptoms of psoriasis. Robinson et al. (1996) found a significant decrease in anxiety and an increase in confidence of facially disfigured people (among whom were people with acne and vitiligo) after a social skills workshop that aimed at improving social interaction skills. Additionally, Ehlers et al. (1995), in their controlled trial, used relaxation therapy with patients with atopic dermatitis and found significant improvement in the skin condition.

Cognitive–behavioural therapy

Cognitive–behaviour therapy (CBT) is a treatment approach that aims to change maladaptive ways of thinking, feeling and behaving through the use of cognitive and behavioural interventions. This model takes the view that it is not situations in and of themselves that are stressful, but rather the perception that one takes of them that makes them so. According to the cognitive model, the beliefs that patients hold about their condition often influence how they cope with and adapt to it. A common feature in the beliefs of people with emotional difficulties is that they have negative and irrational content. These perceptions are often the result of distortions in processing, such as 'cognitive errors' (Beck, 1976, 1993).

CBT focuses on examining and trying to challenge dysfunctional beliefs and appraisals, which may be implicated in a person's low mood or avoidance of certain situations or behaviours. Consequently, targeting cognitions and maladaptive behaviour are the key areas of CBT interventions for facilitating change. According to this approach, beliefs are considered as hypotheses to be tested rather than assertions to be uncritically accepted. Therapist and client take the role of 'investigators' and develop ways to test beliefs, such as 'Others do not like me because of my eczema' or 'I won't be happy anymore because of my vitiligo'. Success at challenging these beliefs involves providing evidence that they are erroneous, and underscored by anxiety and depression (Beck, 1993).

CBT has been successfully applied to various skin conditions. For example, Horne et al. (1989) used cognitive–behavioural therapy along with standard medical treatment in treating three patients suffering with atopic eczema. All three showed a post-treatment reduction in symptom severity, an increase in their ability to control the disorder and a decrease in their reliance on medication. Four controlled studies have also used a cognitive–behavioural approach with psoriasis patients (Price et al., 1991; Zacharie et al., 1996; Fortune et al., 2002; Fortune et al., 2004). Findings have shown adjunctive cognitive–behavioural interventions result in a reduction of psychological distress and in the clinical severity of the condition. Additionally, Papadopoulos et al. (1999b) compared two matched groups of vitiligo patients, one of which received CBT while the other received standard medical treatment alone. Results suggested that patients could benefit from CBT in terms of coping and living with vitiligo. There was also preliminary evidence to suggest that gains made through CBT influences the progression of the condition. Finally, Ehlers et al. (1995) employed CBT with patients with atopic dermatitis and found significant reductions in anxiety, frequency of scratching and itching as well as cortisone use.

Psychoanalytic psychotherapy and hypnosis

Psychoanalytic psychotherapeutic approaches place emphasis in psychodynamics and in particular to unconscious processes. Transference and counter-transference phenomena as well as patients' resistance are all dynamic aspects of the therapeutic relationship and important clinical concepts for this model. The basic goal of this type of therapy is to make the unconscious conscious and to create meaning where there is anxiety or confusion.

The integration of the psychoanalytic approach in dermatology has been realised in some examples of dermatological conditions where patients (such as patients with urticaria or eczema) are not yet aware of a psychogenic factor in their dermatosis. There are case reports in the literature where the use of psychoanalytic psychotherapy led to marked improvements in skin conditions (Van Moffaert, 1992).

Early researchers in psychodermatology experimented with the use of hypnosis (Van Moffaert, 1992). Hypnosis brings about changes in physiological parameters, such as skin conductance, skin temperature and vasomotor reactions all of which can be decisive in the aetiology of skin diseases (Van Moffaert, 1992). Neurodermatitis, chronic urticaria and viral warts are skin diseases with which hypnosis has been successfully used (Barber, 1978).

Group therapy

Group therapy is a mode of intervention that helps individuals with a common problem enhance their social functioning though group exercises. Group members are given the opportunity to share their experiences, feelings and difficulties in a safe atmosphere under the auspices of a group facilitator. Using a combination of instruction, modelling, role-play, feedback and open discussion, members of the group are encouraged to discover more about the interaction process. In most cases 6–12 clients meet with their therapist at least once a week for about 2 hours. Usually groups are organised around one type of problem (such as coping) or type of client (such as psoriasis patients).

Through group interaction, ineffective and immature ways of coping are discouraged, positive attitudes are fostered and feelings, such as loneliness and isolation, that many patients experience, diminish. Moreover, group members can bolster one another's self-confidence and self-acceptance, as they come to trust and value one another, and develop group cohesiveness. Group therapy allows participants to try out new skills in a supportive environment and members learn from one another. Thus this offers features not found in individual treatment.

Various approaches, such as social skills training to group therapy have been tried with patients with skin disorders (Robinson et al., 1996). Patients with chronic skin conditions, such as psoriasis or eczema are known to benefit from group therapy and such therapy has increased their confidence in coping with the disease (Ehlers et al., 1995; Seng & Nee, 1997; Fortune et al., 2002).

Overall, research suggests that psychological treatments lead to improvements in clinical severity of skin condition and reductions in psychological distress. This idea corroborates reports that psychological interventions are useful adjuncts to dermatological treatment in such cutaneous disorders and, when combined, can be considered an effective way of managing patients with such conditions. Skin disease appears to be a complex interplay of biological, psychological and social factors, and treatment should exist within the context of this interplay.

Specifically, CBT is gaining credibility as a psychological treatment in the management of skin condition. Data from the studies reviewed are generally supportive of its efficacy as an approach, which can be used as an adjunct to medical care (Ehlers et al., 1995; Papadopoulos et al., 1999; Fortune et al., 2002, 2004). Findings have shown that cognitive techniques produced reductions in the frequency of cognitions concerning itching, catastrophizing cognitions (Ehlers et al., 1995), and in beliefs about the consequences and the emotional causes of disease, and were maintained at 6 month and at 1-year follow-up. Research has also shown that relaxation is an important component of CBT and it has proved most effective in decreasing anxiety levels among dermatology patients (Ehlers et al., 1995; Zacharie et al., 1996). These data suggest that high anxiety levels often observed in these patients can be reduced with treatment and that treatment effects can be maintained even after a 1-year follow-up.

Recommendations for treatment

The present review has certain treatment implications for the management of people with skin conditions. It underscores the fact that the effects of dermatological conditions permeate much deeper than the skin (Papadopoulos et al., 1999b). Consequently, when treating dermatology patients one needs to take into account the impact that their conditions have on their emotional well-being and quality of life and we should seek to develop therapies that would address these factors.

The recognition that cognition, emotion, behaviour and motives have an impact on skin disorders opens new possibilities regarding assessment and treatment in the field of psychodermatology (Papadopoulos & Bor, 1999). A biopsychosocial model of skin disease enables us to go further than simply acknowledging that multiple systems (psychological, physiological, social, environmental factors) interact to produce states of health and illness by providing evidence for the reciprocity between the body and the mind. In order to understand the psychological consequences of dermatological conditions and to treat them effectively, we need to view the patient holistically. Psychological therapies or counselling can be considered an effective adjunct to medical treatment for various skin disorders.

The use of counselling or therapy in the field of dermatology encompasses the idea that people have the capacity to cope with their difficulties and to grow emotionally. Through this process the patient is encouraged to move towards openness and self-trust as opposed to feeling stuck or invalidated (Papadopoulos & Bor, 1999). Therefore, it is useful firstly to explain the way that counselling can help and secondly to distinguish between the different levels of counselling in order to illustrate the range of activities carried out by clinicians.

How can therapy help in the treatment and management of dermatology patients?

Therapy such as CBT can help dermatology patients to:

- come to terms with their conditions;
- explore treatment options and facilitate decision-making;
- examine difficulties they are experiencing with their condition and gain insight into what factors maintain those difficulties;
- explore and challenge dysfunctional appraisals, beliefs and assumptions;
- identify useful coping strategies;
- facilitate social interaction skills;
- examine issues that may be indirectly linked to the skin condition;
- challenge and cope with anticipatory anxiety and depression.

Group therapy, especially social and assertiveness skills training can help dermatology patients:

- encounter difficulties in social situations;
- discuss their problems with others who can empathise;
- develop a better understanding through the others' experiences of their condition;
- allow members to acquire and develop a variety of skills and put them in practice with other members;
- serve as a means of emotional and social support for skin patients.

Levels of counselling

Information giving (education)

This concerns the provision of factual information and advice about medical conditions, treatments, drug trials, disease prevention and health promotion among others.

Implications counselling

This concerns the discussion with the patient and/or others about the implications of the information received regarding the illness for the individual or his/her family and his/her personal circumstance.

Supportive counselling

In supportive counselling, the emotional consequences of the information and its implications can be identified and addressed in a supportive and caring environment.

Psychotherapeutic counselling: therapy

This focuses on healing, psychological adjustment, coping and problem resolution. Different theoretical approaches involve CBT, psychoanalytic therapy, behaviour therapy, humanistic therapy and others.

Conclusion

This chapter examined the close and complex relationship between psychology and skin disease in an attempt to demonstrate the need for psychological interventions in the treatment of dermatological conditions. Indeed, it has been shown that there is a real need to address psychosocial issues surrounding disfiguring dermatological conditions. The impact skin disease has on the patients' well-being as well as his/her relationship to the outer world can be great and varied. Hence, a major aim of the present chapter was to conceptualise skin disorders as a biopsychosocial phenomenon, which have the ability to exert negative pressures on sufferers and therefore their management calls for a holistic approach.

Although evidence was provided that psychological treatments can be efficacious in addressing them, still much of the research in this area is methodologically flawed. Some studies often have small numbers of patients and some lack appropriate controlled groups. Additionally, as the majority of the research has employed quantitative designs, much of the depth of information regarding patients' beliefs about psychotherapeutic approaches, such as relevance, motivation and expectations is lost. Finally, studies have failed to examine variables, such as length of treatment and treatment at different stages of illness, which can provide more data on the benefits accrued from such approaches.

Therefore, there is a great need for systematic evaluation to determine the treatment efficacy of different approaches to counselling and the development of psychological treatments, which will focus on the unique issues pertaining to dermatology patients. Future research should seek to examine the utility of different modalities for various skin conditions by employing designs that will compare them. Thus, controlled studies should be devised to compare differences between the effectiveness of different psychological treatments as well as varying time and stage of illness. Moreover, future research should seek to address factors, such as motivation, adherence to treatment and treatment expectations. On the whole, it appears that the positive outcome of therapy is dependent on non-specific variables, such as motivation and expectations rather than on specific treatment variables per se (Van Moffaert, 1992). Hence, investigations with less motivated and committed samples need to be considered in order to establish precisely the types of individuals that are likely to benefit from therapeutic services.

In conclusion, the fact that psychological interventions can have important effects on the severity of chronic dermatological disorders offers an exciting prospect for the management of skin patients. Certainly, we have come a long way in our understanding of the relationship between psychological factors and dermatological conditions. More knowledge and education of the public around issues concerning counselling and its effectiveness in dermatological conditions is needed. Prejudicial beliefs about psychological services as well as patients' own psychological difficulties, particularly perceptions of stigmatisation, may impede them from attending such treatments. However, as health professionals we can begin to overcome these obstacles by providing patients with comprehensive information about psychological approaches and helping them to make more effective use of and derive benefits from the psychological interventions available to them. Ultimately, dermatological conditions, like other illnesses, need to be addressed not only in terms of the objective effects of the illness but also in terms of the subjective experience of the patient; it is only through well-researched, methodologically sound psychological techniques that we can ever hope to address that.

REFERENCES

Al-Abadie, M.S., Kent, G.G., & Gawkrodger, D.J. (1994). The relationship between stress and the onset and exacerbation of psoriasis and other skin conditions. *British Journal of Dermatology*, **130**, 199–203.

Barber, T.X. (1978). Hypnosis, suggestions and psychosomatic phenomena: a new look from the stand point of recent experimental studies. *American Journal of Clinical Hypnosis*, **21**, 113–127.

Beck, A. (1976). *Cognitive Therapy and Emotional Disorders*. New York: International Universities Press.

Beck, A. (1993). Cognitive therapy: past, present and future. *Journal of Consulting and Clinical Psychology*, **61**, 194–198.

Cole, W.C., Roth, H.L., & Sachs, L.B. (1988). Group psychotherapy as an aid in the medical treatment of eczema. *Journal of the American Academy of Dermatology*, **18(2)**, 286–291.

Ehlers, A., Stangier, U., & Gieler, U. (1995). Treatment of atopic dermatitis: a comparison of psychological and dermatological approaches to relapse prevention. *Journal of Consulting and Clinical Psychology*, **63(4)**, 624–635.

Fortune, D.G., Richards, H.L., Main, C.J., & Griffiths, C.E.M. (2000). Pathological worrying illness perceptions and disease severity in patients with psoriasis. *British Journal of Health Psychology*, **5**, 71–82.

Fortune, D.G., Richards, H.L., Griffiths, C.E.M., & Main, C.J. (2004). Targeting cognitive–behavioural therapy to patient's implicit model of psoriasis: results from a patient preference controlled trial. *British Journal of Clinical Psychology*, **43**, 65–82.

Fortune, D.G., Richards, H.L., Kirby, B., Bowcock, S., Main, C.J., & Griffiths, C.E.M. (2002). A cognitive–behavioural symptom management programme as an adjunct in psoriasis therapy. *British Journal of Dermatology*, **146**, 458–465.

Ginsburg, J.H. (1995). Psychological and psychophysiological aspects of psoriasis. *Dermatologic Clinics*, **13**(4), 793–804.

Gray, S.G., & Lawlis, G.F. (1982). A case study of pruritic eczema treated by relaxation and imagery. *Psychological Reports*, **51**, 627–633.

Griffiths, C.E.M., & Richards, H.L. (2001). Psychological influences in psoriasis. *Clinical and Experimental Dermatology*, **26**, 338–342.

Gupta, M.A., Schork, N.J., Gupta, A.K., Kirkby, S., & Ellis, C.N. (1993). Suicidal ideation in psoriasis. *International Journal of Dermatology*, **32**, 188–190.

Horne, D.J.L., White, A.E., & Varigos, G.A. (1989). A preliminary study of psychological therapy in the management of atopic eczema. *British Journal of Medical Psychology*, **62**, 241–248.

Hughes, J.E., Barraclough, B.M., Hamblin, L.G., & White, J.E. (1983). Psychiatric symptoms in dermatology patients. *British Journal of Psychiatry*, **143**, 51–54.

Kellett, S., & Gilbert, P. (2001). Acne: A biopsychosocial and evolutionary perspective with a focus on shame. *British Journal of Health Psychology*, **6**, 1–24.

Koblenzer, C.S. (1983). Psychosomatic concepts in dermatology. *Archives of Dermatology*, **119**, 501–512.

Papadopoulos, L., & Bor, R. (1999). *Psychological Approaches to Dermatology.* Leicester, UK: BPS.

Papadopoulos, L., & Walker, C. (2003). *Understanding Skin Problems: Acne, Eczema, Psoriasis and Related Conditions.* West Sussex, UK: Wiley.

Papadopoulos, L., Bor, R., & Legg, C. (1999a). Psychological factors in cutaneous disease: an overview of research. *Psychology, Health & Medicine*, **4**(2), 107–126.

Papadopoulos, L., Bor, R., & Legg, C. (1999b). Coping with the disfiguring effects of vitiligo: A preliminary investigation into the effects of cognitive–behavioural therapy. *British Journal of Medical Psychology*, **10**, 385–396.

Papadopoulos, L., Bor, R., & Legg, C., & Hawk, J.LM. (1998). Impact of life events on the onset of vitiligo in adults: preliminary evidence for a psychological dimension in aetiology. *Clinical and Experimental Dermatology*, **23**, 243–248.

Papadopoulos, L., Bor, R., Walker, C., Flaxman, P., & Legg, C. (2002). Different shades of meaning: Illness beliefs among vitiligo sufferers. *Psychology, Health & Medicine*, **7**(4), 425–433.

Price, M.L., Mottahedin, I., & Mayo, P.R. (1991). Can psychotherapy help with psoriasis? *Clinical and Experimental Dermatology*, **16**, 114–117.

Robinson, E., Rumsey, N., & Partridge, J. (1996). An evaluation of the impact of social interaction skills training for facially disfigured people. *British Journal of Plastic Surgery*, **49**, 281–289.

Seng, T.K., & Nee, T.S. (1997). Group therapy: A useful and supportive treatment for psoriasis patients. *International Journal of Dermatology*, **36**(2), 110–112.

Thompson, A.R., & Kent, G. (2001). Adjusting to disfigurement: processes involved in dealing with being visibly different. *Clinical Psychology Review*, **21**, 663–682.

Thompson, A.R., Kent, G., & Smith, J.A. (2002). Living with vitiligo: dealing with difference. *British Journal of Health Psychology*, **7**, 213–225.

Van Moffaert, M. (1992). Psychodermatology: an overview. *Psychotherapy & Psychosomatics*, **58**, 125–136.

Weinstein, M.Z. (1984). Psychosocial perspectives on psoriasis. *Dermatologic Clinics*, **2**, 507.

Winchell, S.A., & Watts R.A. (1988). Relaxation therapies in the treatment of psoriasis and possible pathophysiologic mechanisms. *Journal of the American Academy of Dermatology*, **18**, 101–104.

Wolpe, J. (1980). Behaviour therapy for psychosomatic disorders. *Psychosomatics*, **21**, 379–385.

Zacharie, R., Oster, H., Bjerring, P., & Kragballe, K. (1996). Effects of psychologic intervention on psoriasis: A preliminary report. *Journal of the American Academy of Dermatology*, **34**, 1008–1015.

9

Research methodology in quality of life assessment

Andrew Finlay

Introduction

The concept of trying to measure the impact that skin disease has on patients' lives has only gained wide acceptance over the past 10 years. Dermatologists have always, presumably, been aware of the devastating effect that skin disease can have upon the lives of their patients, but historically most publications have focused on the pathology of the skin rather than on the subsequent effect on the patient. This chapter will introduce the reasons why measurement methods are needed, review the major techniques that have been described and detail how they are validated. Some recent research findings will be reviewed and current challenges for further research in this area identified.

What is quality of life?

The concept of what constitutes quality of life (QoL) is controversial (Koller & Lorenz, 2002) and whether it can be meaningfully measured even more so. The following attempt at defining QoL emphasises the difficulties in defining what most people feel they instinctively understand: 'Quality of life can be defined as the individual's perception of their position in life, in relation to their goals and to the value-system which they have accepted and incorporated in to their decision-making' (Sartorius, 1993). There is a more limited concept of health-related QoL that is limited to the effects that health or its absence has on life. The World Health Organisation (WHO) has given definitions of and explained how disease can lead to impairment, which leads to disability and which in turn may lead to handicap (WHO, 1980).

Why QoL measurement is important?

There are several reasons why it is important to try to measure the impact of skin disease on QoL. In many health care systems throughout the world, resource allocation to dermatology is inadequate. Thankfully few patients die from their skin disease but this makes it harder to argue for dermatology resources. The use of general QoL measures allows comparison of the major effects of skin diseases with the effects of other non-skin diseases. In clinical research there has traditionally been an emphasis on using clinical signs as outcome measures but QoL measurement gives an additional and patient-orientated outcome assessment, which does not necessarily parallel change in signs. The importance of this distinction has been emphasised by recent work in psoriasis (Sampogna et al., 2004). This study has clearly demonstrated that measurement techniques cluster into two groups, one formed by clinical severity measurements and the other comprising QoL and psychological indexes, stressing the need for more comprehensive assessment. Many pharmaceutical companies are recognising this and adding QoL measurement to clinical drug assessment protocols.

Both clinical services and novel ways to deliver services are required to be audited and in these contexts it is both more practical and more relevant for QoL measures to be used as primary outcome measures. In routine clinical practice, clinicians reach a 'judgement' of how severely individual patients' lives are affected by their skin disease. This information is used in the risk/benefit considerations relating to treatment decisions. Unfortunately clinicians may not be as accurate as they think they are in these assessments and the use of simple QoL measures may be useful to inform some critical decisions, for example where systemic drugs with significant side effects are being considered.

Development of QoL research in dermatology

A 21-question format was suggested in 1970 to record, in a standard way, the impact of skin disease on QoL (Whitmore, 1970). Other suggestions concerning criteria for assessing the impact of permanent skin impairment (Committee, 1970) and systems for wider assessment of disability (Robinson, 1973) were also proposed. The first dermatology disease-specific instrument, the Psoriasis Disability Index (PDI) (Finlay & Kelly, 1985; Kelly & Finlay, 1987) was initially used to assess the impact of hospital admission on disability in patients with psoriasis and has subsequently been used widely (Lewis & Finlay, 2004). The use of validated, standardised general health measures in dermatology, such as the UK Sickness Impact Profile (Finlay et al., 1990) and the Short Form-36 (SF-36) (Nichol et al., 1996) followed in the early 1990s. Several dermatology disease-specific QoL measures for use in acne, psoriasis, atopic dermatitis, alopecia, leg ulcers and others were described during the 1990s and 2000s. It became clear however in the early 1990s that many of the impacts on QoL experienced by patients were similar, whatever may be the nature of the skin disease. What was required were simple measures that could be used across a wide range of different skin diseases. The Dermatology Life Quality Index (DLQI) was created to meet this need (Finlay & Khan, 1994): this measure has since been used very widely internationally (Lewis & Finlay, 2004). Subsequently several other measures, such as Skindex (Chren et al., 1996), the Freiberg Life Quality Assessment (Augustin et al., 2004), Dermatology-Specific QoL (Anderson & Rajagopolan, 1997) and Dermatology QoL Scales (Morgan et al., 1997) have been described for use across all skin diseases in adults.

It is clearly inappropriate for measures designed for adults to be used in children. The specific needs of different age groups were first addressed in 1995 by the Children's DLQI (CDLQI) (Lewis-Jones & Finlay, 1995). Since then the disease-specific measure, the Infants Dermatitis QoL questionnaire (Lewis-Jones et al., 2001), has been described.

There was recognition of the potential value of being able to measure the secondary impact of skin disease on the family in 1998 by the publication of the disease-specific questionnaire the Family Dermatitis Index (Lawson et al., 1998).

An entirely different way of gaining insight into patients' attitudes to their disease is the use of utility questions. This approach seeks to find out the value that patients place on their disease by asking hypothetical questions relating monetary or time equivalents to changes in disease states. This was first used in acne (Motley & Finlay, 1989), in psoriasis (Finlay & Coles, 1995; Zug et al., 1995), and in atopic dermatitis (Finlay, 1996a), further attention is now being given to this approach (Littenberg et al., 2003; Schiffner et al., 2003).

Although QoL questionnaires are now widely used in dermatology for clinical research and audit, they are not yet regularly used in routine clinical work either as outcome measures or to aid clinical decision-taking. It is necessary for the meaning of QoL scores and the meaning of QoL score change to be easily understood by clinicians before these instruments will be widely helpful. This issue is being addressed (Hongbo et al., 2004) but remains an important research challenge in the development of QoL assessment in dermatology.

Methods of creation of measures

It is tempting, but wrong, for health professionals to think that they understand in detail the ways in which their clients' or patients' lives can be affected by their disease. It is essential that this information is sought from patients themselves, the first step in the creation of any system to measure the impact of skin disease on people's lives is to gain this information directly from those affected. This may be by unstructured or structured interview, by seeking information in writing or by using focus groups. Clearly the target audience for the use of the measure must be reflected in the population studied, taking into account age range, sex, language and/or cultural definitions. Some authors of QoL measures also use already published information or seek the views of health care professionals as part of their information gathering exercise. This seems reasonable provided this information is simply to confirm that no aspects have been overlooked (i.e. to validate the primary information gathering from patients); it should not be used as part of the primary information on which to base the proposed measure. Information should continue to be sought from those affected until continuing to interview others is revealing no new information.

Once the body of information has been gathered, very closely related areas of impact on patients' lives need to be merged into single descriptors. By this stage there will still usually be a long list of items that have been identified in this way. The next challenge is to use this information as the basis of a questionnaire tool. There are differing approaches as to how to amalgamate the information into a questionnaire that reflects the reality of the situation from the patients' viewpoint.

One possibility is to identify items which are very closely correlated: one of these items can be discarded in the knowledge that change in the presence or absence of this item will normally be exactly reflected in change in the kept item. This process can be repeated until the number of items reaches a level that is realistic for practical purposes or until no items remain that are correlated closely enough to cut. The problem with this scientifically sound approach is that there is the risk that the acceptability of the final series of items may have reduced comprehensiveness or acceptability for patients. The patient may perceive that the questionnaire reveals a lack of understanding of the subject area as aspects are omitted; their omission being due to close correlation with persisting items.

An alternate approach is less satisfactory from the statistical point of view but may result in greater face validity. The 'long list' of items are classified into various domains so that similar items, for example all those relating to work or to personal relationships, are grouped together. Within each domain the number of items can be reduced by the methods above, thereby at least ensuring a spread of questions viewed by the patient as appropriate. Alternatively the domain groups of questions can be reduced by a subjective approach of coalescing similar items into broader questions that encompass the contributing concepts.

Once a list of questions has been identified a draft questionnaire can be written. The time basis of the questions must be specified: this needs to be short if the instrument is going to be of any value to detect clinical change following intervention.

Validation techniques

The draft questionnaire must be tested on a group of patients to assess comprehensibility and to detect any other obvious flaws. Once changes are made, a second similar exercise needs to be carried out to check the appropriateness of any changes. Once there is an agreed final version a process of internal and external validation can start.

Internal validation of measures attempts, by factor analysis, to establish whether the questions are uni-dimensional and so can legitimately be summarised in a single score, or whether there are independent domains represented in the question structure. Internal consistency should also be determined by means of Cronbach's alpha.

External validation involves establishing test–retest reliability, correlation with other similar existing and previously validated methods, and a process of demonstrating that the new measure is appropriately able to change, reflecting changes in clinical condition.

Test–retest reliability has to be demonstrated to ensure that the format of the questions is such that they are understood clearly and are specific enough so that the same patient will answer the questionnaire in the same way after a short interval. A series of patients with stable disease are asked to complete the questionnaire twice. The interval needs to be short enough to assume that the reality of the patients' life will not have changed, but long enough that it is unlikely that the patient will be able to remember how they answered the first time. This of course involves compromise and intervals of 3–7 days are often chosen.

Construct validity is determined by examining correlation between QoL scores and demographic factors, and other measures used in parallel. Establishing correlation with other existing methods is possible where obvious comparators exist, for example a new disease-specific measure can be compared in the same population with a wider dermatology-specific measure that is likely to encompass many of the concepts of the new measure. It is less easy where an entirely new aspect of QoL is being established, for example when a method for measuring the family impact of atopic dermatitis in children was first proposed (Lawson et al., 1998).

Sensitivity to change is an essential requirement if a measure is to be used as an outcome measure after any intervention, such as a new therapy. There needs to be clarity in the drafting of questions, especially over implicit guidance and a reminder to the reader that the questions relate to the impact of disease over a specific period. The choice of the period will limit the frequency of use of the measure. If, for example, the questions all relate to the patients' experience over the last month, it would not be possible to use the questionnaire to detect, after a week, changes in QoL caused by a rapidly effective new therapy. There should clearly be consistency within the questions over the time period: it is not appropriate to mix questions that relate to the last week, which are sensitive to change, with open ended questions relating to a lifetime experience that are insensitive to change. The ability of a questionnaire to change can be established by using it in a before and after intervention which is known to be very effective in alleviating disease activity.

Methodology available

Over the last 20 years a very wide range of questionnaires have been developed for use in patients with skin disease: the following list is not fully comprehensive, but it includes the majority of the most widely used techniques. Many general health measures have and are being used in dermatology but are not listed here.

Dermatology-specific measures: adults

- Dermatology Life Quality Index (Finlay & Khan, 1994; Lewis & Finlay, 2004)
- Skindex (Chren et al., 1996)
- Dermatology-Specific Quality of Life (Anderson & Rajagopolan, 1997)
- Dermatology Quality of Life Scales (Morgan et al., 1997)
- Freiberg Life Quality Assessment (Augustin et al., 2004)

Dermatology-specific measures: children

- Children's Dermatology Life Quality Index (CDLQI) (Lewis-Jones & Finlay, 1995)
- Children's Dermatology Life Quality Index (CDLQI) (Cartoon version) (Holme et al., 2003)

Disease-specific measures

Psoriasis

- Psoriasis Disability Index (PDI) (Finlay & Kelly, 1987; Lewis & Finlay, 2004)
- Psoriasis Life Stress Inventory (PLSI) (Gupta & Gupta, 1995)
- Salford Psoriasis Index (PSI) (Kirby et al., 2000)
- PSORIQoL (McKenna et al., 2003)

Atopic dermatitis

- Infant's Dermatitis QoL Index (IDQOL) (Lewis-Jones et al., 2001)
- Dermatitis Family Impact (DFI) Questionnaire (Lawson et al., 1998)
- QoL Index for Atopic Dermatitis (QoLIAD) (Whalley et al., 2004)

Acne

- Acne Disability Index (Motley & Finlay, 1989)
- Cardiff Acne Disability Index (Motley & Finlay, 1992)
- Assessment of the Psychological and Social Effects of Acne (Layton, 1994)
- Acne-Specific Quality of life Questionnaire (Acne-QoL) (Girman et al., 1996; Martin et al., 2001)
- Acne Quality of Life Scale (Gupta et al., 1998)

Other disease-specific measures
- Chronic venous insufficiency (FLQA) (Augustin et al., 1997)
- Skin disease in human immunodeficiency virus (HIV)-infected patients (HIV-DERMDEX) (Aftergut et al., 2001)
- Melasma (MELASQOL) (Balkrishnan et al., 2003)
- Alopecia (WAA-QOL) (Dolte et al., 2000)
- Scalp dermatitis (Scalpdex) (Chen et al., 2002)

Critical reviews of methodology

In view of the proliferation of QoL measures in dermatology, several authors have sought to identify and review published measures against various criteria (Finlay & Ryan, 1996; Finlay, 1997; de Korte et al., 2002, 2004).

Use of methods

QoL measures have been used widely in dermatology over the last decade. Examples of the uses to which such measures can be put will focus largely on recent experience of the DLQI, which was developed by our group.

Therapeutics

There is now a widespread use by pharmaceutical companies of QoL measures as additional outcome measures in clinical trials of new drugs. Recent examples include a study from Germany that demonstrated that use of topical pimecrolimus cream in adults with atopic dermatitis results in major improvement of QoL, as well as in standard clinical parameters (Meurer et al., 2004). Similar improvement was seen in a study from Korea (Won et al., 2004) using topical tacrolimus in adults and children with atopic dermatitis.

Health service research

There are many modalities of therapy for psoriasis and great variation in methods offered in different health care systems. In some Scandinavian countries, patients are offered climate therapy that involves spending treatment time at a more southern sunny latitude. It is appropriate that these methods should be evaluated: a recent study of psoriasis patients from Norway treated in Turkey (Mork et al., 2004) demonstrated statistically significant improvement in severity and QoL scores.

Epidemiology: national surveys

The DLQI is well suited for use in large-scale epidemiological studies as it is easily completed without the need for detailed instructions. Used in a recent survey of patients with ichthyosis in Sweden (Ganemo et al., 2004), significant differences of QoL scores were seen between major ichthyosis types. QoL measures can be used sequentially in long-term studies to assess the longer-term impact of disease, as illustrated by the recent study in Australia (Jenner et al., 2004). Patients with atopic dermatitis were assessed in a 1-year prospective study: this study highlighted substantial financial and other effects on patients.

Patient disease interaction

Although women over-report symptoms in non-dermatologic disease, gender dependent differences in patients' perception of skin disease are poorly described. A study from Sweden (Holm et al., 2004) has examined these differences in the self-reported morbidity of patients with atopic dermatitis. Normally visible areas of atopic dermatitis appear to affect women significantly more than men.

Recent further DLQI validation studies

It is important that general dermatology measures should be demonstrated to be valid in specific diseases and in different cultures. In two multicentre studies (Lennox & Leahy, 2004) in the USA of 418 and 439 patients with chronic idiopathic urticaria, the DLQI was demonstrated to be valid, reliable and a clinically useful outcome measure.

A recent study has demonstrated similar good validity in the use of the DLQI in 70 patients with vitiligo in Iran (Aghaei et al., 2004). A significant difference was demonstrated in the personal relationship domain sub-scores between patients with involvement of covered-only areas, and those with involvement of both covered and uncovered areas.

A cultural validation of the DLQI Polish translation demonstrated good reliability and internal consistency (Szepietowski et al., 2004), allowing this tool to now be used in Poland. There are at least 22 language translations of the DLQI now available.

Psychological symptoms and compliance

The relationship of QoL of patients to acne severity, anxiety and depression were examined in a study in Turkey (Yazici et al., 2004). This study of 61 patients demonstrated an increased risk of depression in patients compared to controls. The greater the impairment of QoL due to acne, the greater the level of anxiety and depression. The relationship of QoL impairment to psychological symptoms was also demonstrated in a study from Denmark of 333 dermatology outpatients, 172 inpatients and 293 matched controls (Zachariae et al., 2004). High impairment of QoL as measured using the DLQI was the main predictor of psychological symptoms.

A study of 100 patients with hand eczema used both the DLQI and the generic questionnaire, the SF-36 (Wallenhammar et al., 2004). There was a high correlation between the instruments for physical health, but it was considered that in this group of patients the SF-36 measured mental health better than the DLQI.

Insights into the problems of compliance of dermatology patients with treatment can be gained by using QoL measures. Two hundred and one patients with psoriasis were interviewed and re-examined 3 months later to assess actual treatment use and compare this with expected use (Zaghloul & Goodfield, 2004a). There was an inverse relationship between medication adherence and impairment of QoL: patients with facial disease and more extensive disease had lower medication adherence. This information will encourage appropriate strategies to try to enhance adherence in groups who can now be identified as being at high risk of poor adherence. The same group has demonstrated that outpatients with psoriasis under the direct supervision of a consultant demonstrated better adherence and had lower DLQI scores (i.e. less impairment of QoL) than similar patients attending the nurse-led clinic (Zaghloul & Goodfield, 2004b).

Influences affecting QoL

A postal questionnaire study in Sweden used the DLQI to measure QoL and record possible influences on perceived QoL (Uttjek et al., 2004). The strongest indicators for impaired QoL were large disease extent and joint symptoms: another indicator was withdrawal from medical treatment due to distance from treatment facilities.

Further research challenges

The need for further research in the area of QoL measurement in dermatology were addressed in a UK All Party Parliamentary Group report (Working Party, 2003). 'It was considered that funding should be made available for research into the creation and use of methodology to measure the impact of skin diseases on individuals. Further research is required into the long-term consequences on major life decisions and the influence this has on the development and QoL of individuals. Funding should be made available for research on the psychological and social impact of rare diseases, which is often overlooked in favour of more prevalent conditions.' The explicit setting of objectives by this group will hopefully act as an encouragement to funding of such research.

QoL measures are now being used frequently in dermatology research but, 20 years since they were first introduced into dermatology, they are very seldom ever used in the routine clinical setting. As outlined above, clinicians may not be accurate in estimating the extent to which their patients are affected by their skin disease: having a quick, easy and accurate way to measure this would have the potential to inform clinical decision-taking. One reason that QoL measures are not used in this way is that it is not easy for clinicians to understand the scores and relate them to the clinical situation. Although this information is now becoming available for the DLQI (Hongbo et al., 2004), such data is not yet available for other measures. The validated banding of DLQI scores with simple descriptive terms will allow physicians, and indeed perhaps, in time, patients to use this questionnaire to guide decision-taking. More data is required, however, to understand the link between score bands and types of decision that are taken. There is preliminary data relating to psoriasis, which suggests that in routine clinical practice there is a relationship between decision type and patient QoL impairment (Katagumpola et al., 2004). More information is required relating to the most common inflammatory diseases. It will be necessary to seek similar data for other measures before they are likely to find a place in routine clinical use.

Therapy for inflammatory skin diseases, which is already complex, is likely to become much more so over coming years. Currently there is a major upheaval in the possibilities for treating severe psoriasis, with the advent of several systemic biologics. As part of the development of these drugs, QoL data has been gathered, mainly using the DLQI. Protocols incorporating levels of QoL impairment may be helpful to guide clinicians over appropriate use of these and existing drugs, and need to be developed.

Up to now, attempts at defining disease activity in dermatology have focused on formulae for the quantification of signs and symptoms (Finlay, 1996b). It is now becoming accepted that from the patients' viewpoint, impact on QoL is of equal importance to the level of disease activity, and QoL measures have the potential to allow integration of assessment of QoL into standard assessment protocols defining disease activity. One example is the proposal (Finlay, 2005) to define Severe Current Psoriasis by the Rule of Tens: Current Severe Psoriasis = Body Surface Area affected (BSA) >10% *or* Psoriasis Area and Severity Index (PASI) >10 *or* DLQI >10. Relatively simple concepts such as this will emphasise the importance of QoL in patient assessment: other disease severity concepts incorporating QoL information are needed for use in other inflammatory skin diseases.

The vast majority of QoL research published in dermatology relates to adults. Although there are several general dermatology measures and several hundred publications describing their use, the information relating to QoL research in children is much less comprehensive. In contrast to the very widespread use of the adult DLQI (Lewis & Finlay, 2004), there are currently only 13 full articles and 21 abstracts describing the use of the CDLQI, the first children-specific dermatology measure (www.ukdermatology.co.uk., 2004). There are considerable difficulties in designing QoL measures for children, both because of rapidly changing levels of children's understanding and because of changing daily activities as children develop. There are important challenges in this field.

Although assessment of QoL in children has not received as much attention as the subject in adults, there are other important age groups that have been even less attended to. Teenagers and adolescents have lifestyles and concerns that are often distinct from those of children or adults. Their special needs are sometimes overlooked and new methods to assess the impact of skin disease on this age group are required. The very elderly may also have distinctly different lives with, for example, a greater reliance on others for support and a value-system which, tempered by wisdom and age, assigns less importance to some aspects of life and greater importance to others. In dermatology as in other branches of medicine, different risk/benefit analyses need to take place when taking clinical decisions in the very elderly. For example, when using methotrexate the risk of long-term side effects will be of much lower importance. The ability to gain further insight into patient's attitudes to QoL in this group has the potential to contribute to more appropriate decision-taking.

The special QoL issues experienced by patients with skin disease are not always adequately reflected by general health measures, such as the SF-36 or EuroQoL-5, though there is some evidence that in some circumstances their use may add information not captured by dermatology-specific measures (Wallenhammar et al., 2004). In the main, the experience of patients with skin disease was not specifically considered when general health tools were constructed. Unfortunately from the point of view of dermatology, methods of value comparison between different disease types used by national bodies with influence over resource allocation may involve the use of these general measures, for example when constructing quality adjusted life years (QALY) data. This may, in the long term, be to the disadvantage of patients with skin disease. Therefore, there is an additional research challenge to enmesh the data from disease-specific tools such as the DLQI with other general tools in order to reflect to the maximum the impact of skin diseases compared to other non-skin disease.

A long-term goal of research into QoL in dermatology is to reach a point where it is normal daily clinical practice to take into account QoL information in routine decision-taking.

Declaration of interest

Professor A Y Finlay is joint copyright owner of the DLQI, CDLQI, ADI, CADI, IDQOL and DFI. His department receives some income from their use. For more information about these measures: www.dermatology.org.uk

REFERENCES

Aftergut, K., Carmody, T., & Cruzm, P.R. (2001). Use of the HIV-DERMDEX quality-of-life instrument in HIV-infected patients with skin disease. *International Journal of Dermatology*, **40**, 472–484.

Aghaei, S., Sodaifi, M., & Jafari, P., et al. (2004). DLQI scores in vitiligo: reliability and validity of the Persian version. *BMC Dermatology*, **4**, 8.

Anderson, R.T., & Rajagopalan, R. (1997). Development and validation of a quality of life instrument for cutaneous diseases. *Journal of the American Academy of Dermatology*, **36**, 41–50.

Augustin, M., Dieterle, W., & Zschocke, I., et al. (1997). Development and validation of a disease-specific questionnaire on the quality of life of patients with chronic venous insufficiency. *VASA*, **26**, 291–301.

Augustin, M., Lange, S., Wenninger, K., Seidenglanz, K., Amon, U., & Zschocke, I. (2004). Validation of a comprehensive Freiburg Life Quality Assessment (FLQA) core questionnaire and development of a threshold system. *European Journal of Dermatology*, **14**, 107–113.

Balkrishnan, R., McMichael, A.J., & Camacho, F.T., et al. (2003). Development and validation of a health-related quality of life instrument for women with melasma. *British Journal of Dermatology*, **149**, 572–577.

Committee on rating of mental and physical impairment; guides to evaluation of permanent impairment. (1970). *Journal of American Medical Association*, **211**, 106–112.

Chen, S.C., Yeung, J., & Chren, M-M. (2002). Scalpdex a quality of life instrument for scalp dermatitis. *Archives of Dermatology*, **138**, 803–807.

Chren, M-M, Lasek, R.J., Quinn, L.M., Mostow, E.N., & Zyzanski, S.J. (1996). Skindex, a quality-of-life measure for patients with skin disease: reliability, validity and responsiveness. *Journal of Investigative Dermatology*, **107**, 707–713.

de Korte, J., Mombers, F.M.C., & Sprangers, M.A.G., et al. (2002). The suitability of quality of life questionnaires for psoriasis research: a systematic literature review. *Archives of Dermatology*, **138**, 1221–1227.

de Korte, J., Sprangers, M.A.G., & Mombers, F.M.C., et al. (2004). Quality of life in patients with psoriasis: a systematic literature review. *Journal of Investigative Dermatology Symposium Proceedings*, **9**, 140–147.

Dolte, K.S., Girman, C.J., & Hartmaier, S., et al. (2000). Development of a health-related quality of life questionnaire for women with androgenic alopecia. *Clinical and Experimental Dermatology*, **25**, 637–642.

Finlay, A.Y. (1996a). Measures of the effect of severe atopic eczema on quality of life. *Journal of the European Academy of Dermatology and Venereology*, **7**, 149–159.

Finlay, A.Y. (1996b). Measurement of disease activity and outcome in atopic dermatitis. *British Journal of Dermatology*, **135**, 509–515.

Finlay, A.Y. (1997). Quality of life measurement in dermatology: a practical guide. *British Journal of Dermatology*, **136**, 305–314.

Finlay, A.Y. (2005). Current severe psoriasis and the rule of tens. *British Journal of Dermatology*, **152**, 861–867.

Finlay, A.Y., & Coles, E.C. (1995). The effect of severe psoriasis on the quality of life of 369 patients. *British Journal of Dermatology*, **132**, 236–244.

Finlay, A.Y., & Kelly, S.E. (1985). Psoriasis: an index of severity. *Scottish Medical Journal*, **30**, 266.

Finlay, A.Y., & Kelly, S.E. (1987). Psoriasis – an index of disability. *Clinical and Experimental Dermatology*, **12**, 8–11.

Finlay, A.Y., & Khan, G.K. (1994). Dermatology Life Quality Index (DLQI): a simple practical measure for routine clinical use. *Clinical and Experimental Dermatology*, **19**, 210–216.

Finlay, A.Y., & Ryan, T.J. (1996). Disability and handicap in dermatology. *International Journal of Dermatology*, **35**, 305–311.

Finlay, A.Y., Khan, G.K., Luscombe, D.K., & Salek, M.S. (1990). Validation of Sickness Impact Profile and Psoriasis disability Index in psoriasis. *British Journal of Dermatology*, **123**, 751–756.

Ganemo, A., Sjoden, P.O., & Johansson, E., et al. (2004). Health-related quality of life among patients with ichthyosis. *European Journal of Dermatology*, **14**, 61–6.

Girman, C.J., Hartmaier, S., & Thiboutot, D., et al. (1996). Evaluating health-related quality of life in patients with facial acne: development of a self-administered questionnaire for clinical trials. *Quality of Life Research*, **5**, 481–490.

Gupta, M.A., & Gupta, A.K. (1995). The Psoriasis Life Stress Inventory: a preliminary index of psoriasis-related stress. *Acta Dermato-Venereologica*, **75**, 240–243.

Gupta, M.A., Johnson, A.M., & Gupta, A.K. (1998). The development of an acne quality of life scale: reliability, validity and relation to subjective acne severity in mild to moderate acne vulgaris. *Acta Dermato-Venereologica (Stockh)*, **78**, 451–456.

Holm, E.A., Esmann, S., & Jemec, G.B.E. (2004). Does visible atopic dermatitis affect quality of life more in women than in men? *Gender Medicine*, **1(2)**, 125–130.

Holme, S.A., Mann, I., Sharpe, J.L., Dykes, P.J., Lewis-Jones, M.S., & Finlay, A.Y. (2003). The Childrens' Dermatology Life Quality Index: validation of the cartoon version. *British Journal of Dermatology*, **148**, 285–290.

Hongbo, Y., Thomas, C.L., Harrison, M.A., Salek, M.S., & Finlay, A.Y. (2004). Translating the science of quality of life into practice: what do Dermatology Life Quality Index scores mean? *British Journal of Dermatology*, **151 (Suppl. 68)**, 46.

Jenner, N., Campbell, J., & Marks, R. (2004). Morbidity and cost of atopic eczema in Australia. *Australasian Journal of Dermatology*, **45**, 16–22.

Kelly, S.E., & Finlay, A.Y. (1987). Psoriasis – an index of disability. *Clinical and Experimental Dermatology*, **12**, 8–11.

Koller, M., & Lorenz, W. (2002). Quality of Life; a deconstruction for clinicians. *Journal of the Royal Society of Medicine*, **95**, 481–488.

Katagumpola, R.P., Hongbo, Y., & Finlay, A.Y. (2004). The relationship between patient-rated quality of life and clinicians' management decisions in psoriasis – a prospective study. *Journal of Investigative Dermatology*, **123(2)**: A70.

Kirby, B., Fortune, D.G., & Bhushan, M., et al. (2000). The Salford Psoriasis Index: an holistic measure of psoriasis severity. *British Journal of Dermatology*, **142**, 728–732.

Lawson, V., Lewis-Jones, M.S., Finlay A.Y., Reid, P., & Owens, R.G. (1998). The family impact of childhood atopic dermatitis: the Dermatitis Family Impact Questionnaire. *British Journal of Dermatology*, **138**, 107–113.

Layton, A.M. (1994). Psychological assessment of skin disease. *Interfaces in Dermatology*, **1**, 9–11.

Lennox, R.D., & Leahy, M.J. (2004). Validation of the Dermatology Life Quality Index as an outcome measure for urticaria-related quality of life. *Annals of Allergy Asthma and Immunology*, **93**, 142–146.

Lewis, V.J., & Finlay, A.Y. (2004). Ten years experience of the Dermatology Life Quality Index (DLQI). *Journal of Investigative Dermatology Symposium Proceedings*, **9**, 140–147.

Lewis, V.J., & Finlay, A.Y. (2004). Two decades' experience of the Psoriasis Disability Index. *Dermatology,* **151**(**68**), 50–51.

Lewis-Jones, M.S., & Finlay, A.Y. (1995). The Children's Dermatology Life Quality Index (CDLQI): initial validation and practical use. *British Journal of Dermatology*, **132**, 942–949.

Lewis-Jones, M.S., Finlay, A.Y., & Dykes, P.J. (2001). The Infants' Dermatitis Quality of Life Index. *British Journal of Dermatology*, **144**, 104–110.

Littenberg, B., Partilo, S., & Licata, A., et al. (2003). Paper standard gamble: the reliability of a paper questionnaire to assess utility. *Medical Decision Making*, **23**, 480–488.

Martin, A.R., Lookingbill, D.P., & Botek, A., et al. (2001). Health-related quality of life among patients with facial acne – assessment of a new acne-specific questionnaire. *Clinical and Experimental Dermatology*, **26**, 380–385.

McKenna, S.P., Cook, S.A., & Whalley, D., et al. (2003). Development of the PSORIQoL, a psoriasis-specific measure of quality of life designed for use in clinical practice and trials. *British Journal of Dermatology*, **149**, 323–331.

Meurer, M., Fartasch, M., & Albrecht, G., et al. (2004). Long-term efficacy and safety of pimecrolimus cream 1% in adults with moderate atopic dermatitis. *Dermatology*, **208**, 365–372.

Morgan, M., McCreedy, R., Simpson, J., & Hay, R.J. (1997). Dermatology quality of life scales: a measure of the impact of skin diseases. *British Journal of Dermatology*, **136**, 202–206.

Mork, C., Ozek, M., & Wahl, A.K. (2004). Treatment of leisure? Climate therapy of patients with psoriasis and psoriatic arthritis. *Tidsskr Nor Laegeforen*, **124**, 60–62.

Motley, R.J., & Finlay A.Y. (1989). How much disability is caused by acne? *Clinical and Experimental Dermatology*, **14**, 194–198.

Motley, R.J., & Finlay, A.Y. (1992). Practical use of a disability index in the routine management of acne. *Clinical and Experimental Dermatology*, **17**, 1–3.

Nichol, M.B., Margoilies, J.E., Lippa, E., Rowe, M., & Quell, J. (1996). The application of multiple quality of life instruments in individuals with mild-to-moderate psoriasis. *Pharmacoeconomics*, **10**, 644–653.

Robinson, H.M. (1973). Measurement of impairment and disability in dermatology. *Archives of Dermatology*, **108**, 207–209.

Sampogna, F., Sera, F., & Abeni, D., et al. (2004). Measures of clinical severity, quality of life, and psychological distress in patients with psoriasis: a cluster analysis. *Journal of Investigative Dermatology*, **122**, 602–607.

Sartorius, N. (1993). A WHO method for the assessment of health-related quality of life. In: S.R. Walker, & R.M. Rosser (Eds.), *Quality of Life Assessment: Key Issues in the 1990s*. London: Kluwer Academic Publishers, pp. 201–207.

Schiffner, R., Schiffner-Rohe, J., Gerstenhauer, M., Hofstadter, F., Landthaler, M., & Stolz, W. (2003). Willingness to pay and time trade-off: sensitive to changes of quality of life in psoriasis patients. *British Journal of Dermatology*, **148**, 1153–1160.

Szepietowski, J., Salomon, J., & Finlay, A.Y., et al. (2004). Dermatology Life Quality Index (DLQI): Polish version. *Dermatologia Kliniczna*, **6**, 63–70.

Uttjek, M., Dufaker, M., & Nygren, L., et al. (2004). Determinants of quality of life in a psoriasis population in northern Sweden. *Acta Dermato-Venereologica*, **84**, 37–43.

Wallenhammar, L-M., Nyfjall, M., & Lindberg, M., et al. (2004). Health-Related quality of life and hand eczema – a comparison of two instruments, including factor analysis. *Journal of Investigative Dermatology*, **122**, 1381–1389.

Whalley, D., McKenna, S.P., & Dewar, A.L., et al. (2004). A new instrument for assessing quality of life in atopic dermatitis: international development of the Quality of life Index for Atopic Dermatitis (QoLIAD). *British Journal of Dermatology*, **150**, 274–283.

Whitmore, C.W. (1970). Cutaneous impairment, disability and rehabilitation. *Cutis*, **6**, 106–112.

Won, C.H., Seo, P.G., & Park, Y.M., et al. (2004). A multicenter trial of the efficacy and safety of 0.03% tacrolimus ointment for atopic dermatitis in Korea. *Journal of Dermatological Treatment*, **15**, 30–34.

Working Party. (2003). *Report on The Enquiry into the Impact of Skin Diseases on People's Lives.* All Party Parliamentary Group on Skin, London.

World Health Organisation. (1980). *International classification of impairments, disabilities, and handicaps.* Geneva.

www.ukdermatology.co.uk (2004) (accessed 9 October 2004).

Yazici, K., Baz, K., & Yazici, A.E., et al. (2004). Disease-specific quality of life is associated with anxiety and depression in patients with acne. *JEADV*, **18**, 435–439.

Zachariae, R., Zachariae, C., & Ibsen, H.H.W., et al. (2004). Psychological symptoms and quality of life of dermatology outpatients and hospitalised dermatology patients. *Acta Dermato-Venereologica*, **84**, 205–212.

Zaghloul, S.S., & Goodfield, M.J.D. (2004a). Objective assessment of compliance with psoriasis treatment. *Archives of Dermatology,* **140**, 408–414.

Zaghloul, S.S., & Goodfield, M.J.D. (2004b). The influence of nurse education clinics as a supplementary technique on compliance in psoriasis. *British Journal of Dermatology*, **151**(**Suppl. 68**), 51.

Zug, K.A., Littenberg, B., & Baughman, R.D., et al. (1995). Assessing the preferences of patients with psoriasis. *Archives of Dermatology*, **131**, 561–568.

10

Psychodermatology in context

Carl Walker

Introduction

There has been a considerable increase, in the last two decades, in cosmetic surgery and dieting as well as the profile of the fashion and cosmetic industry. The 'appearance industry' is a multi-million pound business aimed at selling beauty products to the widest possible market and this has served to increase the pressure that many people feel to conform to unreachable standards in physical aesthetics. Particularly in the Western world, we see adverts that project the agenda that 'attractive people are popular, happy, successful, interesting and are often loved and worshipped' (Papadopoulos & Walker, 2003). This is particularly acute when looking at adverts for facial washes and scrubs for acne that intentionally contrast the relative social successes of individuals with and without a given skin disease. Of course, cosmetic and physical perfection are rarely associated with those experiencing cutaneous conditions and so people with dermatological illnesses are often left feeling minimised as people. Modern adverstising can promote just the kind of messages that psychological health professionals try to minimise; that is, to put your life on hold until the skin disease clears and to feel less worth than those around you with clear skin. Skin disease patients can, understandably, be highly sensitive to the social significance of their actions and appearance, and the development of beliefs about their disease are influenced by the information they receive from their culture (Papadopoulos & Bor, 1999).

As this book shows, the field of psychodermatology touches upon a relatively wide number of areas both academically and with regard to the effects of skin disease on patients. This concluding chapter draws together some of the research findings to date within a theoretical framework that emphasises our understanding about the importance of the beliefs that patients hold about their skin disease. An anecdotal illustration of the effect that skin disease can have on a sufferer is provided in order to frame some of the aforementioned theory of earlier chapters within an everyday, colloquial context. This chapter also touches upon the issues facing psychodermatology as a multidiscipline and the role of psychodermatology in the future, emphasising the implementation of the growing body of psychological knowledge available to health professionals.

A theoretical framework for skin disease: what do patients know about their own skin disorder?

The psychology of the dermatology patient is a relatively under-researched area and so suffers from a relative lack of clarity. We have substantially covered the psychosocial effect that skin disease can have upon an individual and their social system but, just as important, is the way that the patient represents their illness. Understanding these dermatological illness representations might play a fundamental role in understanding treatment compliance, behavioural adaptation, impact upon relationships, the way a person copes with the often episodic nature of the disease and a number of other crucial aspects of the skin disease experience discussed throughout the book. Yet, so little is still known about how people actually conceptualise their disease along a number of cognitive dimensions. The literature indicates that there are generally higher levels of psychological distress amongst people with skin conditions but crucially, there is also evidence to suggest that there is considerable individual variation. Several studies have found only a weak association between disease severity and psychological functioning (Finlay et al., 1990; Fortune et al., 1997, 2002) and, as previously stated, lay beliefs about the origin and maintenance of skin conditions abound and may differ across cultures. Beliefs within the domain of illness representations have been shown to be influential in medical help-seeking. The use of outpatient services, disease-related distress, disability, avoidance and the use of concealment behaviours are all the common social anxiety-related adjustment strategies, and depend heavily on the way that people represent their illness.

Indeed, the mother–child relationship may be affected by a child with a skin condition and the considerable variation between mothers with respect to how they respond to a skin condition depends on factors related to the appearance of the baby but also the mother's own beliefs and attitudes concerning skin diseases and physical appearance (Walters, 1997). Some mothers can react to the illness by exhibiting overprotection and overindulgence of the child whereas others can feel that the condition impinges on their ability to bond with their child and can lead to great distress. Furthermore, the recent development of the Illness Perception Questionnaire for children shows that the way that children represent their skin condition is also of considerable importance (Walker et al., 2004).

Schober and Lacroix (1991) argue that modern contemporary illness models, as the explanatory framework of health and illness, are fundamentally based in the

Hippocratic–Galenic medicine of classic Greek antiquity. Today it is thought that identity (symptoms), cause, consequences, cure and timeline appear to be the major attributes of illness representations (Leventhal et al., 1997), and that they are a loosely organised set, defining the objective problem or associated danger.

Each feature of a great many patients' representations of illness can generate strong affective reactions. These reactions can be provoked either by an abstract label (e.g. vitiligo) or by the concrete component (depigmentation of the skin) of the representation and we can distinguish three broad sources of information that people draw upon for the elaboration of illness representations (Leventhal et al., 1984). These are:

- The generalised pool of illness information current in the culture.
- Social communication or information obtained in direct contact with other people, particularly practitioners.
- The individual's personal illness experience. The local culture of the family and medical care system, the mass media and the openness of other patients as points of comparison as well as the individual's own private experience of disease and its treatment.

As touched upon earlier, Leventhal et al. (1984) identified four principal attributes that appear common to many illness representations.

Identity

Variables that identify the presence or absence of the illness: Skin diseases can be identified by symptoms such as pain and itching, concretely by signs like sores or bleeding and by the use of abstract labels such as eczema or psoriasis. Identity is important because the meaning and interpretation of a symptom can influence the way the person addresses the symptom. Should a patient erroneously apply the label of skin cancer to a white lesion on their skin, this could precipitate a different response than were they to attribute the lesion as a rash or an injury. This is particularly important in the domain of help-seeking.

Consequences

This pertains to the perceived consequences of the disease, physically and emotionally, socially and economically. Individuals who have pessimistic beliefs as regards the health risk that their condition poses may be less likely to seek treatment and this could be particularly salient depending on the gravity of their condition.

Causes

Perceived causes of the disease: This can take a wide range of forms including causes due to the individual's own behaviour (i.e. scratching, poor diet), environmental pathogens (bacteria or viruses) or genetic factors. Chronic, episodic illnesses such as psoriasis and vitiligo tend that patients can often create their own illness beliefs as regards events, behaviours and substances that exacerbate their condition, and this can lead to curious and sometimes dangerous reactions. For instance, the mistaken belief that vitiligo is caused by white foods could cause the parent of the vitiliginous child to ban certain essential foods from the child's diet. The consequences of this action could have negative long-term effects on the child's generic health.

Timeline

This attribute concerns the perceived time frame for the development of the condition or threat. Time frames run through all aspects of illness representations and can be crucial with respect to the way that patients label and conceptualise the illness. A patient with newly diagnosed psoriasis may assume from the knowledge that they have gained that the condition is episodic and hence should remit in the near future. This could prompt a set of short-term avoidance behaviours designed to conceal the condition. However, a failure to repigment could result in these avoidant and concealment behaviours becoming ingrained and permanent.

Lau and Hartmann (1983) added curability or controllability to this group of attributes and these attributes can play a crucial role in the way that a person with a skin disease represents and reacts to their condition. There can be a tendency for people to develop and rely on their own lay intuitions as to how their disease started, the factors that exacerbate the disease and how they can best treat their condition (Leventhal et al., 1984; Weinman et al., 1996; Affleck et al., 1997). The importance of understanding patients' illness cognitions cannot be underestimated, and as we will see in the next section, they can play an important role in the way that patients react to instances of felt and actual stigma.

The importance of personal illness beliefs and stigma regarding skin disease

To some extent, skin conditions are unique from many other diseases in so far as they are often visible to others. Through much of this book we have focused on felt stigma, that is, the stigma perceived by the sufferer. While skin disease and some of the associated behaviours and coping strategies can have a tendency to reinforce cognitive conceptualisations of the condition that can be overtly negative and biased, skin disease patients also experience actual or enacted stigma.

While felt stigma is of utmost importance to both skin disease patients and health professionals, instances of enacted stigma, where the respondent believed that he or she was being treated abnormally in some way, may be common in often visible skin conditions. Indeed, Ginsberg et al. (1993) point out that in one study, 19% of the patients reported incidents of blatant rejection in which they were explicitly asked to leave a restaurant, swimming pool, health club or hairdressers and there is emerging evidence that many people hold negative implicit attitudes (attitudes not subject to alteration in response to social desirability) towards people with visible skin conditions (Grandfield et al., 2004).

Many people with skin diseases have experienced their condition when they were young or at least some of their beliefs regarding skin diseases would have initially developed at a young age and so the reaction of child peers can be of great importance. Children and adolescents are especially vulnerable to the influence of television and magazines because they do not necessarily reflect on the messages communicated to them (Papadopoulos & Walker, 2003). This is especially important for children who may not have personal experience of those who look physically different and rely heavily on the television to 'fill-in' the gaps in their knowledge. Many children do not understand skin disease and disfigurement in the same context that adults do and so they often behave inappropriately in response to the disfigured individual. Children are not socialised to the same extent as adults and so their treatment of other children with skin disease can be considerably worse than the treatment that adult skin disease sufferers may receive. The case of enacted stigma can be particularly painful for children with skin disease since, unlike adults, young children are less inhibited in their approach to their peers. They will often stare openly at a child who looks different, and will sometimes tease and bully the child with specific regard to their condition. If we understand how pervasive myths regarding skin disease are with adults then we can see that knowledge amongst children will be even more inaccurate. Indeed, a great deal of adults who experienced skin disease as a child have very traumatic recollections regarding their interaction with their peers (Richardson, 1997).

Although there has been sufficient research to suggest that those with impaired appearance do engender negative reactions (Papadopoulos et al., 1999), very little speculation has taken place concerning the reasons for this. Robinson et al. (1996) suggests three possible answers, they are:

- Negative reactions could arise from the just world hypothesis; that is, people generally get what they deserve in life and a person's disfigurement will serve as punishment for previous transgressions.
- Avoidance may be maintained due to people being unsure how to approach and behave around people who are visibly different.
- People may fear contagion due to a lack of understanding about the condition.

Updike (1990) has written eloquently about the enacted stigma of the psoriasis sufferer. He believed that the tendency for people without skin disease to turn away from people with skin disease or to feel disconcerted stems from a fleeting identification with the person who is afflicted. The affected person symbolises our own vulnerability and imperfection, our defensiveness and lack of autonomy. Updike speculates that we turn away from those who remind us of our own inherent humanity and vulnerability.

The relationship between felt stigma and enacted stigma is very important in the context of the skin disease experience. For psychological health professionals to be able to help skin disease patients with body image and self-esteem problems, the relationship between these two factors and the way that the patient processes acts of enacted stigma are very important. Like most acts of physical and verbal violence, the perceived responsibility for acts of enacted stigma can determine lifestyle choices for many skin disease patients. Here, a good example of the way that a person frames their condition in the context of Leventhal et al. (1984) illness representations model can have particular prescience. The attribution of causality with regard to unpleasant and aggressive remarks about a person's skin can lead to many believing that they are responsible for this treatment because they have 'taken ownership' of this skin disease. This may result from the belief in common myths on causality ('I eat the wrong foods', 'I do not wash properly'), beliefs about the skin disease that have carried over from childhood (such as those originating from the circumstances that they were engaged in when their condition first developed) or because of personal cognitive factors which make them more vulnerable to self-blame. Whatever the reason, some skin disease patients can take responsibility for their condition and allow the stigma generated from remarks, and staring to penetrate and disable them in a way that it may not do for others. In conjunction with the appearance industry's concentration on visual perfection, enacted stigma can act to utterly disable and dismay many sufferers of skin conditions to an extent that they allow beliefs about their skin to dictate the way that they value themselves as a whole. This can spread to other aspects of a person's life that influence their self-esteem, aspects that may not at first seem related to their beliefs about their skin disease. Many people obtain a sense of value in themselves from a number of sources such as job achievement, academic achievement and close relationships, among others, and all of these sources of esteem can mean little to someone whose feelings concerning their skin have pervaded the very essence of the way that they represent themselves.

Indeed the extent to which patients will react to their condition by representing themselves in the context of their disease or believing that others represent them in the context of their disease can be influenced by the cognitive representations of the self formed and reinforced over many years.

Linville (1987) proposed that individual differences in vulnerability to stress are influenced by cognitive conceptualisations of the self; more specifically due to the differences in the complexity of self-representations. Cognitive complexity is defined as a greater number of self-aspects and the maintenance of greater distance between self-aspects. The author states that for those who manage to generate greater complexity, negative events are likely to impact less as they are confined to a smaller portion of the self-representation. Indeed this logic is also used in models of cognitive–behavioural therapy (CBT) when the impact of negative events and indeed negative cognitions are reduced. The author showed that greater self-complexity acted as a moderator of depressions and illness when people were under high stress.

If, for a given reason or set of circumstances in the past, early beliefs about the self were formed with little compartmentalisation of self-aspects then a negative focus on the body could create an experience that activates negative feelings and negative beliefs about the self as a whole. That is, the self as a husband, as a lover, as a father, an employee, a friend; as an intelligent, valuable human being.

Skin disease and psychotherapy: an example of how psychology can help

The importance of the way that an illness is represented cognitively has been shown to be important in a number of aspects of living with a skin disease. Thus if we assume that illness schemata are implied in behavioural and coping strategies then faulty schemata may result in dysfunctional responses. Illness schemata represent learned patterns of perception and cognition, and can be extremely resistant to change. To alter maladaptive illness and/or personal representations and to change ineffective coping strategies, one must understand a patients' current belief structures as regards the way in which they perceive the different facets of their illness and the way that they represent how they look and feel. This understanding then has to be used to generate new experiences that will correct the existing system. For example, when appraisals change the definition of a health problem and make a tractable problem appear intractable, or when they damage confidence in one's sense of control over the disease and its impact on their life, there will be a diminution or elimination of motivation to maintain curative or disease-limiting behaviours (Papadopoulos & Walker, 2003).

The experience of adult skin disease patients can be extremely varied and some people may be relatively unaffected by a wide spread of the condition whereas others can be devastated by a relatively small, minimal and invisible lesion. The reason for this disparity in the psychological and physiological properties (or concrete and abstract aspects, as conceptualised in Leventhal's terminology) of the condition concerns the notion that disfiguring skin diseases do not affect psychosocial adjustment in a vacuum. People develop representations of their illness in conjunction with their previous knowledge and beliefs concerning their self-worth, their image of their body and their previous knowledge of skin diseases, in order to create a relatively unique disease concept.

The case of Jake

The example below of Jake[1], a 29 year-old psoriasis sufferer who developed the condition 10 years ago is instructive:

'I had always been a real sports fan for as long as I can remember. Through my teens I had been involved in county and school teams at cricket, rugby and football. That changed when I started to develop psoriasis on my legs in my late teens. I became really aware of it and self-conscious and couldn't face going in the showers in case team-mates saw it and felt repulsed. I knew that they would think it was contagious. I certainly did at first, you know, like I was a leper or something so rather than let this happen I gradually dropped out of sport, certainly team sport anyway. I suppose the same thing happens when the weather gets warm in the summer. My psoriasis is more progressive now and so I always cover it up, regardless of the weather. This can mean that I'm often uncomfortable in the summer heat and feel almost permanently vigilant but at least this disease doesn't get seen by others.

It's a shame that I can't play sport any more but I suppose I could have worse diseases, even if I do worry a lot about my psoriasis spreading again.'

The above vignette from one of the participants who came to take part in a London Metropolitan University research therapy programme is informative of the issues that these patients can face. As soon as Jake developed the disease, a number of precepts were automatically activated, which created the framework for Jake to contextualise his condition and the effect that it would have on his everyday life. Automatic assumptions regarding the repulsed attitudes of friends, team-mates and the general public concerning contagion and leprosy were untested and unchallenged but these cognitions became settled into a pattern of contextualising future social episodes regarding his disease. An automatic picture of 'what others thought' was created in conjunction with ideas of what the condition represented. This consideration of the social impact of the disease vitiated Jake's quality of life, serving to influence the clothes that Jake wore and hone a sense of vigilance with regards to the visibility of his condition. The lack of reality testing and creation of possible alternative thoughts had led to a seemingly unequivocal acceptance of his inability to play sport, an activity that he had previously enjoyed immensely.

This example touches upon the importance of the cognitive architecture that can frame beliefs about the disease, its social context and the way that patients can allow aspects of a disfiguring illness to exert a measure of control over their life. As

---

[1] The name of this participant has been changed to protect his identity and permission to use his account was secured.

mentioned in Chapter 8, CBT allows us to challenge and change these thoughts and beliefs. It allows participants to be located outside of their own automatic thoughts and actions and hence be able to reflect on the way that they may have profoundly limited aspects of their everyday life and that this need not be the case. CBT can work by altering deeply held schematic conceptualisations of the self and the disease such that patients are not confined by the often untested representations that they construct.

Of crucial importance in many cases, and with particular relevance to Jake is why he developed these concepts of his disease and why he initially believed that friends and colleagues, not to mention strangers, would automatically react so negatively to the presence of his psoriasis. Jake developed psoriasis as a man with 19 years of experience that had informed and fashioned a cognitive structure that worked to guide him in the different challenges that he faced. Another skin disease patient may not have created the automatic thoughts that Jake did and it is this history that plays such an important role in influencing and guiding our reactions.

The body as aesthetic object

Individual CBT can allow a therapist to study Jake's view of himself and the premium he placed on the aesthetic value of his body. Many schemas are laid down in the early years of living and those that act maladaptively can integrate later experience within this maladaptive context. They may work to create such ramifications as feelings of social anxiety, shame and poor self-esteem.

Rather than focus on the functional aspects of the body, the body can be viewed from an aesthetic perspective and self-criticism can act as part of a campaign to judge the self by impossibly high standards. The number of self-aspects in which a patient engages and the extent to which they compartmentalise cognitive aspects of the self can profoundly influence feelings of self-worth in the presence of a given social context. CBT often works to separate the self from the disease, which in many cases is the paramount issue since the disease can come to represent the self in an aesthetic context. Working with patients to re-emphasise aspects of the self that are not dependent on the body and to help them to realise that others often do not base their judgement of the patient on their body and specifically, their skin disease, can be a crucial aspect of the therapeutic process.

Psychology and treatment

As touched upon above, attention has increasingly been given to the therapeutic benefits that might derive from psychological interventions. As discussed in Chapter 8, the research literature has documented psychological interventions for a number of cutaneous conditions (Van Moffaert, 1992; Papadopoulos & Bor, 1999), and an array of techniques and approaches have been adopted within this context. These include psychoanalysis and hypnosis (Gray & Lawlis, 1982) behavioural techniques (Wolpe, 1980) and CBT (Papadopoulos et al., 1999). These interventions have been shown to produce clinically significant improvements (Van Moffaert, 1992) and have helped people to improve their quality of life (Papadopoulos et al., 1999). Group therapy has also proved beneficial, allowing the loneliness and isolation that many patients experience to be diminished. Self-confidence and acceptance can be developed within a trusting and cohesive atmosphere.

The use of counselling or therapy in the field of dermatology encompasses the idea that people have the capacity to cope with their problems and address them. In the context of dermatology this often means being able to separate themselves from the vagaries of their condition, to allow their self-concept and quality of life to be developed independent of the episodic nature or severity and visibility of their disease.

There is, however, a great need for further evaluation of these different approaches in order to maximise the practical benefits that health professionals can deliver to this population and future research should focus on methodologically valid, comparative paradigms to achieve this. Much of the research in this field has taken the form of single case studies or group trials with small samples or inadequate control comparisons. Outcome measures have been crude and sometimes involved only the undocumented observations of one clinician. It is also important to note that the vast majority of work has come from Western countries and therefore the results found may not be generalisable to other cultures. Further research should focus on this aspect of psychodermatological treatment. Much work has also tended to be retrospective and hence limited in the conclusions that can be drawn (Papadopoulos et al., 1999). Finally, theoretical coherence should always be an aim of research such that a meaningful and useful framework can be created on which to base future research and clinical treatment.

The professional perspective

The benefits of psychological treatment for some skin disease patients are well known but there can be stigma associated with using psychological therapy and it is important to understand patients' beliefs and knowledge concerning this treatment. That said, patients approaching health professionals today are arguably more informed and sophisticated in their understanding of medicine than ever before and are often dissatisfied with traditional medical therapies. They often actively seek alternative approaches and adjuncts to standard treatment. Fried (2002) believes that health professionals within the discipline, be they psychiatrists,

paediatricians, nurses, social workers or other mental health specialists, may benefit by being referred to as 'skin emotional specialists'. This may improve patient
likelihood of accepting a psychological referral.

Of course the education of patients with skin disease is of great importance, but
we must also bear in mind that different health professionals have different knowledge bases also. Generally speaking, dermatologists and dermatology professionals
are medically trained and as such may not have the necessary expertise in the psychosocial aspects of the disease as well as the developmental implications of children's health knowledge. In order to adequately inform patients, we have to ensure
that dermatology professionals are familiar with the growing literature on the
psychosocial aspects of dermatology.

Clinicians have an enormous responsibility, not only in the treatment of dermatoses, but in the way that the patient develops the illness representations of their
condition. Those who are apprehensive of incorporating psychological approaches
within their treatment framework should reflect on the consequences of their rigid
adherence to a solely medical approach. This could lead to patients developing
fixed and erroneous beliefs in a solely somatic illness.

Psychodermatology: the multidiscipline

As mentioned in the introduction, this text is intended to provide material of interest for a range of health professionals, including psychologists, psychiatrists, general
practitioners, nurses, dermatologists and any other professionals who work with
dermatology patients. Indeed this multidisciplinary readership is the key context
behind the creation of the book. We intend this book to have sampled the practical
and theoretical expertise of many different health professionals such that cross-
disciplinary misunderstanding is minimised. An emphasis has been given to mental
health professionals working in the field since it is this area in which little is known.

We wish to allow health professionals a little more confidence when encountering scenarios within their practice that may fall outside their immediate realm of
expertise but yet still may be a crucial part of the psychodermatological experience.
This could be a dermatologist understanding in greater detail the way that children
and their parents are affected by a given disease or perhaps a psychiatrist learning
more about the psychoneuroimmunology of the skin disease.

The field of psychodermatology has suffered from a distinct demarcation in
publication coverage between the physiological and psychosocial research. Few
dermatology practitioners are regular subscribers to health psychology journals and
it is unlikely that many psychologists keep informed of the latest work in dermatology
journals but a way to bridge this gap is crucial. Journals like 'Dermatology and
Psychosomatics' are beginning to play a crucial role in research cross-fertilisation

in such a fashion that it becomes available to as wide an academic and professional readership as is possible and we hope that this text has contributed to playing a similar role.

A framework for the future

An important issue for future research concerns the strengthening of the links between theoretical and empirical studies on the ways in which people cope with health threats and research concerning illness representations. There is a gap to be found in these two areas and since the concept of implicit health models was developed in the context of understanding coping processes, it would make sense to attempt to bridge this gap (Croyle, 1992).

Regarding the treatment of the issues that we know are important with respect to the skin disease experience, any monoform treatment of psychodermatoses is bound to be ineffective for many patients, regardless of whether this is psychologically or medicinally based. A mixed approach is necessary which allows an appropriate, idiosyncratic and combined therapy for the individual patient. As mentioned, the lack of a clear relationship between skin disease severity and psychosocial morbidity suggests that this idiosyncratic approach is of paramount importance. Many skin disease sufferers have suggested that more training is needed to support clinicians in listening to patients and to help them develop their empathy, especially for patients with scratching difficulties.

Finally, one of the difficulties with working in the field is the realisation that the government, health professionals and voluntary agencies often fail to work together as closely as they might to ensure that services are consistent across the country. This would benefit all patients by improving the information and support that they require. It should however be noted that there is plenty of hope for a more positive future for psychodermatology. During a substantial research programme, we have found many dermatological health professionals with a passion to do whatever is possible to help to advance their discipline with regard to meeting the challenges of the future. This is exhibited by the recent creation of the inaugural UK Psychodermatology Research Group. These positive attitudes to research, allied to work such as that contained within this book suggests that we will move more effectively towards addressing the needs of the patients within our field.

REFERENCES

Affleck, C., Tenner, H., Croog, S., & Levine, S. (1997). Causal attribution, perceived benefits and morbidity after a heart attack: an 8-year study. *Journal of Consulting and Clinical Psychology*, **55**, 29–35.

Croyle, R.T. (1992). Appraisal of health threats: Cognition, motivation, and social comparison. *Cognitive Therapy and Research*, **16(2)**, 165–182.

Finlay, A.Y., Khan, G.K., Luscombe, D.K., & Salek, M.S. (1990). Validation of Sickness Impact Profile and Psoriasis Disability Index in psoriasis. *British Journal of Dermatology*, **123**, 751–756.

Fortune, D.G., Main, C.J., O'Sullivan, T.M., & Griffiths, C.E.M. (1997). Quality of life in patients with psoriasis: the contribution of clinical variables and psoriasis-specific stress. *British Journal of Dermatology*, **137**, 755–760.

Fortune, D.G., Richards, H.L., Griffiths, E.M., & Main, C. (2002). Psychological stress, distress and disability in patients with psoriasis: consensus and variation in the contribution of illness perceptions, coping and alexithymia. *British Journal of Clinical Psychology*, **41**, 157–174.

Fried, R.G. (2002). Non-pharmacologic Treatments in Psychodermatology. *Dermatologic Clinics*, **20(1)**, 177–185.

Grandfield, T., Thompson, A., & Turpin, G. (2004). An attitudinal study of responses to dermatitis using the implicit association test. *Poster presented at the Annual British Psychological Society Conference*, April, 2004.

Gray, S.G., & Lawlis, G.F. (1982). A case study of pruritic eczema treated by relaxation and imagery. *Psychological Reports*, **51**, 627–633.

Linville, P.W. (1987). Self-complexity as a cognitive buffer against stress-related illness and depression. *Journal of Personality and Social Psychology*, **2(4)**, 663–676.

Lau, R.R., & Hartman, K.A. (1983). 'Common sense representations of common illnesses'. *Health Psychology*, **2(March)**, 167–185.

Leventhal, H., Nerenz, D.R., & Steele, D.J. (1984). Illness representations and coping with health threats. In: A. Baum, S.E. Taylor, & J.E. Singer (Eds), *Handbook of Psychology and Health*. Hillsdale, NJ: Erlbaum.

Leventhal, H., Benyamini, Y., Brownlee, S., Diefenbach, M., Leventhal, E.A., Patrik Miller, L., & Robitaille, C. (1997). Illness representations: Theoretical foundations. In: K.J. Petrie, & J.A. Weinman (Eds), *Perceptions of Health and Illness*. Amsterdam: Harwood Academic Publishers.

Papadopoulos, L., & Bor, R. (1999). *Psychological Approaches to Dermatology*. BPS Books. Leicester, England.

Papadopoulos, L., & Walker, C.J. (2003). *Understanding Skin Problems*. John Wiley & Sons Ltd. Chichester.

Papadopoulos, L., Bor, R., & Legg, C. (1999). Coping with the disfiguring effects of vitiligo: a preliminary investigation into the effects of cognitive–behavioural therapy. *British Journal of Medical Psychology*, **72(3)**, 385–396.

Richardson, J. (1997). Chapter 10. In: R. Lansdown, N. Rumsey, E. Bradbury, T. Carr, & J. Partridge (Eds), *Visibly Different: Coping with Disfigurement*. Oxford: Butterworth-Heinemann.

Robinson, E., Rumsey, N., & Partridge, J.P. (1996). An evaluation of the impact of social interaction skills training for facially disfigured people. *British Journal of Plastic Surgery*, **49**, 281–289.

Schober, R., & Lacroix, J.M. (1991). Lay illness models in the enlightenment and the 20th Century: Some historical lessons. In: J.A. Skelton, & R.T. Croyle (Eds), *Mental Representations in Health and Illness*. New York: Springer Verlag.

Updike, J. (1990). *Self Consciousness Memoirs*. London: Penguin Books.

Van Moffaert, M. (1992). Psychodermatology: an overview. *Psychotherapy and Psychosomatics*, **58**, 125–136.

Walters, E. (1997). Problems faced by children and families living with visible difference. In: R. Lansdown, N. Rumsey, E. Bradbury, T. Carr, & J. Partridge (Eds), *Visibly Different: Coping with Disfigurement*. Oxford: Butterworth-Heinmann.

Walker, C., Papadopoulos, L., & Anthis, L. (2004). The IPQ as a reliable measure of illness beliefs for adult acne patients. *Psychology, Health & Medicine* (in press).

Weinman, J., Petrie, K.J., Moss-Morris, R., & Horne, R. (1996). The illness perception questionnaire: a new method for assessing the cognitive representation of illness. *Psychology and Health*, **11**, 431–445.

Wolpe, J. (1980). Behaviour therapy for psychosomatic disorders. *Psychosomatics*, **21**, 379–385.

Index